Integrins and Ion Channels

ADVANCES IN EXPERIMENTAL MEDICINE AND BIOLOGY

Editorial Board:
NATHAN BACK, *State University of New York at Buffalo*
IRUN R. COHEN, *The Weizmann Institute of Science*
ABEL LAJTHA, *N.S. Kline Institute for Psychiatric Research*
JOHN D. LAMBRIS, *University of Pennsylvania*
RODOLFO PAOLETTI, *University of Milan*

Recent Volumes in this Series

Volume 666
PATHOGEN-DERIVED IMMUNOMODULATORY MOLECULES
Edited by Padraic G. Fallon

Volume 667
LIPID A IN CANCER THERAPY
Edited by Jean-François Jeannin

Volume 668
SUPERMEN1
Edited by Katalin Balogh and Attila Patocs

Volume 669
NEW FRONTIERS IN RESPIRATORY CONTROL
Edited by Ikuo Homma and Hiroshi Onimaru

Volume 670
THERAPEUTIC APPLICATIONS OF CELL MICROENCAPSULATION
Edited by José Luis Pedraz and Gorka Orive

Volume 671
FRONTIERS IN BRAIN REPAIR
Edited by Rahul Jandial

Volume 672
BIOSURFACTANTS
Edited by Ramkrishna Sen

Volume 673
MODELLING PARASITE TRANSMISSION AND CONTROL
Edited by Edwin Michael and Robert C. Spear

Volume 674
INTEGRINS AND ION CHANNELS: MOLECULAR COMPLEXES
AND SIGNALING
Edited by Andrea Becchetti and Annarosa Arcangeli

A Continuation Order Plan is available for this series. A continuation order will bring delivery of each new volume immediately upon publication. Volumes are billed only upon actual shipment. For further information please contact the publisher.

Integrins and Ion Channels
Molecular Complexes
and Signaling

Edited by

Andrea Becchetti, PhD
Department of Biotechnology and Biosciences, University of Milano-Bicocca
Milan, Italy

Annarosa Arcangeli, MD, PhD
Department of Experimental Pathology and Oncology, University of Florence
Florence, Itlay

Springer Science+Business Media, LLC
Landes Bioscience

Springer Science+Business Media, LLC
Landes Bioscience

Copyright ©2010 Landes Bioscience and Springer Science+Business Media, LLC

All rights reserved.
No part of this book may be reproduced or transmitted in any form or by any means, electronic or mechanical, including photocopy, recording, or any information storage and retrieval system, without permission in writing from the publisher, with the exception of any material supplied specifically for the purpose of being entered and executed on a computer system; for exclusive use by the Purchaser of the work.

Printed in the USA.

Springer Science+Business Media, LLC, 233 Spring Street, New York, New York 10013, USA
http://www.springer.com

Please address all inquiries to the publishers:
Landes Bioscience, 1002 West Avenue, Austin, Texas 78701, USA
Phone: 512/ 637 6050; FAX: 512/ 637 6079
http://www.landesbioscience.com

The chapters in this book are available in the Madame Curie Bioscience Database.
http://www.landesbioscience.com/curie

Integrins and Ion Channels: Molecular Complexes and Signaling, edited by Andrea Becchetti and Annarosa Arcangeli. Landes Bioscience / Springer Science+Business Media, LLC dual imprint / Springer series: Advances in Experimental Medicine and Biology.

ISBN: 978-1-4419-6065-8

While the authors, editors and publisher believe that drug selection and dosage and the specifications and usage of equipment and devices, as set forth in this book, are in accord with current recommendations and practice at the time of publication, they make no warranty, expressed or implied, with respect to material described in this book. In view of the ongoing research, equipment development, changes in governmental regulations and the rapid accumulation of information relating to the biomedical sciences, the reader is urged to carefully review and evaluate the information provided herein.

Library of Congress Cataloging-in-Publication Data

Integrins and ion channels : molecular complexes and signaling / edited by Andrea Becchetti, Annarosa Arcangeli.
 p. ; cm. -- (Advances in experimental medicine and biology ; 674)
Includes bibliographical references and index.
ISBN 978-1-4419-6065-8
 1. Integrins. 2. Ion channels. 3. Cellular signal transduction. I. Becchetti, Andrea, 1963- II. Arcangeli, Annarosa. III. Series: Advances in experimental medicine and biology ; v. 674.
 [DNLM: 1. Integrins--metabolism. 2. Ion Channels--metabolism. 3. Signal Transduction--physiology. W1 AD559 v.674 2010 / QU 55.7 I612 2010]
 QP552.I55I5795 2010
 571.7'4--dc22
                    2010001223

PREFACE

Interdisciplinarity is more often invoked than practised. This is hardly surprising, considering the daunting vastness of modern biology. To reach a satisfactory understanding of a complex biological system, a wide spectrum of conceptual and experimental tools must be applied at different levels, from the molecular to the cellular, tissue and organismic. We believe the multifaceted regulatory interplay between integrin receptors and ion channels offers a rich and challenging field for researchers seeking broad biological perspectives. By mediating cell adhesion to the extracellular matrix, integrins regulate many developmental processes in the widest sense (from cell choice between differentiation and proliferation, to tissue remodeling and organogenesis). Rapidly growing evidence shows that frequent communication takes place between cell adhesion receptors and channel proteins. This may occur through formation of multiprotein membrane complexes that regulate ion fluxes as well as a variety of intracellular signaling pathways. In other cases, cross talk is more indirect and mediated by cellular messengers such as G proteins. These interactions are reciprocal, in that ion channel stimulation often controls integrin activation or expression. From a functional standpoint, studying the interplay between integrin receptors and ion channels clarifies how the extracellular matrix regulates processes as disparate as muscle excitability, synaptic plasticity and lymphocyte activation, just to mention a few. The derangement of these processes has many implications for pathogenesis processes, in particular for tumor invasiveness and some cardiovascular and neurologic diseases.

This book provides a general introduction to the problems and methods of this blossoming field. It also presents a series of essays on cellular models that have been studied in particular depth. Chapter 1 gives a brief historical background, summarizes the elements of integrin structure and outlines the main biological problems that involve signal transduction between the cell adhesion machinery and ion channels. In Chapter 2, Chiara Di Resta and Andrea Becchetti provide a primer to the structure and physiology of the most relevant ion channel types, which should be useful to readers with a molecular and cell biological background. In the last introductory chapter, Sara Cabodi, Paola Di Stefano, Maria del Pilar Camacho

Leal, Agata Tinnirello, Brigitte Bisaro, Virginia Morello, Laura Damiano, Giusy Tornillo, and Paola Defilippi survey recent views about intracellular signaling triggered by integrin activation, with special emphasis on tyrosine phosphorylation cascades and the relationship with growth factors and cytokines.

The subsequent two chapters review current technology for studying the molecular complexes formed by integral membrane proteins. In particular, Olivia Crociani reviews the main current biochemical and biomolecular strategies, such as the two-hybrid system, the in vitro binding assays and some modern chemical labeling techniques for subsequent optical detection. The latter capture even the weak or transient interactions that are so typical of cellular processes. Alessio Masi, Riccardo Cicchi, Adolfo Carloni, Francesco Saverio Pavone, and Annarosa Arcangeli focus instead on the complementary biophysical methods, such as Förster resonance energy transfer. These not only can provide independent support to the results obtained with biochemical methods, but are invaluable for studying the dynamics, and thus the physiology, of protein-protein interaction.

The final chapters constitute a series of more specific contributions about a few thoroughly studied experimental systems. Margaret Colden-Stanfield illustrates how different types of macrophage K^+ channels, such as inward rectifiers and delayed outward rectifiers, are modulated by cell adhesion. These processes have a role in cell activation and differentiation and thus point to interesting implications for the patophysiology of proliferation and activation of immune cells. These cell types, and blood cells in general, have been the first to be studied from the present book's perspective. Therefore they include some of the best characterized experimental models. The relevance of these studies for the biology of cancer cells is especially addressed by Serena Pillozzi and A. Arcangeli, who mostly expand on the modulatory crosstalk between integrins and the voltage-dependent hERG1 K^+ channel. In several cell lines, membrane complexes containing hERG1, integrin subunits and other proteins, are correlated with neoplastic transformation and could offer novel targets for anti-neoplastic therapy. Another broad field in which the interplay between ion currents and cell adhesion has important physiological roles is cell motility and muscle contraction. Peichun Gui, Jun-Tzu Chao, Xin Wu, Yan Yang, George E. Davis, and Michael J. Davis describe how voltage-gated Ca^{2+} channels and calcium-activated K^+ channels are regulated by integrin-triggered phosphorylation cascades, in vascular smooth muscle. Authors suggest that the myogenic tone and the vascular response to vessel wall injury-remodeling depends on the balance of the integrin-mediated effects on these types of channels. Finally, available evidence also points to interesting modulatory relationships between integrins and ligand-gated channels, particularly glutamate and nicotinic receptors. These recent developments are reviewed by Raffaella Morini and A. Becchetti, who discuss these topics in relation to the development of the central nervous system and synaptic plasticity. The final chapter is devoted to survey what is known about the role of integrins and ion channels in cell migration. This is a relatively unexplored field that we believe merits more intensive research, considering not only the general implication for developmental processes, but also the widespread pathological relevance in processes such as neuronal circuit remodeling, wound healing, and the metastatic progression.

Andrea Becchetti, PhD
Department of Biotechnology and Biosciences
University of Milano-Bicocca
Milan, Italy

Annarosa Arcangeli, MD, PhD
Department of Experimental Pathology and Oncology
University of Florence
Florence, Itlay

ABOUT THE EDITORS...

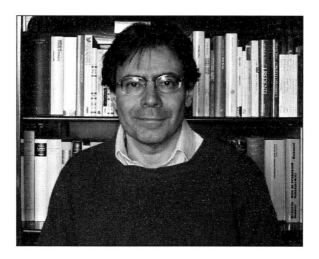

ANDREA BECCHETTI, PhD, is a Professor of General, Comparative and Cellular Physiology at the Department of Biotechnology and Biosciences of the University of Milano-Bicocca, Italy. After receiving his academic degrees at the University of Milan, he has spent prolonged research sojourns at the Department of General Pathology of the University of Florence, Italy, the Department of Physiology at Emory University in Atlanta, Georgia, USA, the Department of Physiological Sciences of the University of Newcastle upon Tyne, UK, and the Biophysics Sector of the International School for Advanced Studies (ISAS-SISSA), in Trieste, Italy.

His current research interests include the role of ion channels in cell adhesion and proliferation, the nicotinic modulation of synaptic transmission in the mammalian cerebral cortex and the pathogenesis of sleep-related epileptic forms linked to mutant human nicotinic receptors. Andrea Becchetti is a member of the Society of General Physiologists, Biophysical Society, Society for Neuroscience and the Italian Physiological Society.

ABOUT THE EDITORS...

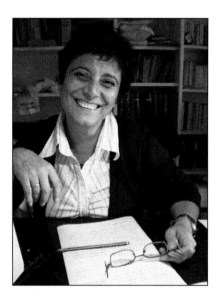

ANNAROSA ARCANGELI, MD, PhD is a Professor of General Pathology and Immunology at the Department of Experimental Pathology and Oncology of the University of Firenze (Florence, Italy). She is the Scientific Director of the Laboratory of Genetic Engineering for the Production of Animal Models of the University of Firenze. After receiving her MD degree at the University of Firenze, she spent several research sojourns at the Department of Physiology of the University of Milano, at the Institut d'Embriologie Cellulaire et Moleculaire, Nogent sur Marne, Paris, France and at the MRC-LMB Centre of Cambridge, UK. Her main research interests include the role of ion channels, in particular potassium channels, in the regulation of different aspects of tumor cell behaviour, including the cross talk with adhesion receptors, as well as the identification of ion channels as novel targets for cancer therapy. Annarosa Arcangeli is a member of the Italian Society of Pathology, the Association of Cell Biology and Differentiation (ABCD), the American Society of Hematology.

PARTICIPANTS

Simona Aramu
Molecular and Biotechnology Center
Department of Genetics Biology
  and Biochemistry
University of Torino
Torino
Italy

Annarosa Arcangeli
Department of Experimental Pathology
  and Oncology
University of Florence
Florence
Italy

Andrea Becchetti
Department of Biotechnology
  and Biosciences
University of Milano-Bicocca
Milan
Italy

Brigitte Bisaro
Molecular and Biotechnology Center
Department of Genetics Biology
  and Biochemistry
University of Torino
Torino
Italy

Sara Cabodi
Molecular and Biotechnology Center
Department of Genetics Biology
  and Biochemistry
University of Torino
Torino
Italy

Adolfo Carloni
European Laboratory for Non-Linear
  Spectroscopy (LENS)
University of Florence
Florence
Italy

Jun-Tzu Chao
Department of Medical Pharmacology
  and Physiology
School of Medicine
University of Missouri
Columbia, Missouri
USA

Riccardo Cicchi
European Laboratory for Non-Linear
  Spectroscopy (LENS)
University of Florence
Florence
Italy

Margaret Colden-Stanfield
Department of Physiology
Morehouse School of Medicine
Atlanta, Georgia
USA

Olivia Crociani
Department of Experimental Pathology
  and Oncology
University of Florence
Florence
Italy

Laura Damiano
Molecular and Biotechnology Center
Department of Genetics Biology
  and Biochemistry
University of Torino
Torino
Italy

George E. Davis
Department of Medical Pharmacology
  and Physiology
School of Medicine
University of Missouri
Columbia, Missouri
USA

Michael J. Davis
Department of Medical Pharmacology
  and Physiology
School of Medicine
University of Missouri
Columbia, Missouri
USA

Paola Defilippi
Molecular and Biotechnology Center
Department of Genetics Biology
  and Biochemistry
University of Torino
Torino
Italy

Maria del Pilar Camacho Leal
Molecular and Biotechnology Center
Department of Genetics Biology
  and Biochemistry
University of Torino
Torino
Italy

Chiara Di Resta
Department of Biotechnology
  and Biosciences
University of Milano-Bicocca
Milano
Italy

Paola Di Stefano
Molecular and Biotechnology Center
Department of Genetics Biology
  and Biochemistry
University of Torino
Torino
Italy

Peichun Gui
Department of Medical Pharmacology
  and Physiology
School of Medicine
University of Missouri
Columbia, Missouri
USA

Alessio Masi
Department of Experimental Pathology
  and Oncology
University of Florence
Florence
Italy

Virginia Morello
Molecular and Biotechnology Center
Department of Genetics Biology
  and Biochemistry
University of Torino
Torino
Italy

Raffaella Morini
Department of Biotechnology and
  Biosciences
University of Milano-Bicocca
Milano
Italy

Serena Pillozzi
Department of Experimental Pathology
  and Oncology
University of Florence
Florence
Italy

Participants

Daniele Repetto
Molecular and Biotechnology Center
Department of Genetics Biology
  and Biochemistry
University of Torino
Torino
Italy

Francesco Saverio Pavone
European Laboratory for Non-Linear
  Spectroscopy (LENS)
University of Florence
Florence
Italy

Agata Tinnirello
Molecular and Biotechnology Center
Department of Genetics Biology
  and Biochemistry
University of Torino
Torino
Italy

Giusy Tornillo
Molecular and Biotechnology Center
Department of Genetics Biology
  and Biochemistry
University of Torino
Torino
Italy

Yan Yang
Department of Medical Pharmacology
  and Physiology
School of Medicine
University of Missouri
Columbia, Missouri
USA

Xin Wu
Department of Systems Biology
  and Translational Medicine
College of Medicine
Texas A&M Health Science Center
College Station, Texas
USA

CONTENTS

1. INTEGRIN STRUCTURE AND FUNCTIONAL RELATION WITH ION CHANNELS 1
Annarosa Arcangeli and Andrea Becchetti

Abstract 1
Introduction 1
Fundamentals of Integrin Structure 2
Physiological and Pathological Implications: An Outline of Current Trends 5
Conclusion 6

2. INTRODUCTION TO ION CHANNELS 9
Chiara Di Resta and Andrea Becchetti

Abstract 9
Introduction 9
The Physiology of Ion Channels 10
Ion Channel Types Involved in Integrin-Mediated Signaling 13
Conclusion 19

3. BIOCHEMICAL METHODS TO STUDY THE INTERACTIONS BETWEEN INTEGRINS AND ION CHANNELS 23
Olivia Crociani

Abstract 23
Introduction 24
Yeast Two-Hybrid Screening 24
Affinity-Based Screening: IP Assays 26
Pull-Down Assay 27
Photoaffinity Labeling Techniques for Studying Transient Protein-Protein Interaction 28
Far Western Blot Analysis (Far WB) 29
High-Throughput Protein-Protein Interaction Analysis, Followed by Validation of Candidate Interactors through Different Experimental Approaches 29
Conclusion 30

4. OPTICAL METHODS IN THE STUDY OF PROTEIN-PROTEIN INTERACTIONS 33

Alessio Masi, Riccardo Cicchi, Adolfo Carloni, Francesco Saverio Pavone, and Annarosa Arcangeli

Abstract 33
Introduction 34
Förster Resonance Energy Transfer: The "Molecular Ruler" 34
Intensity Versus Lifetime: Two Ways to Measure FRET 36
Total Internal Reflection Fluorescence Microscopy (TIRFM) and Imaging
  of Membrane Proteins 38
Antibody-Based Versus Fusion Protein-Based FRET: Principles 38
Antibody-Based Versus Fusion Protein-Based FRET: Advantages
  and Disadvantages 39
Application of Optical Methods to the Study of Integrins and Ion Channels 40
Conclusion 41

5. INTEGRINS AND SIGNAL TRANSDUCTION 43

Sara Cabodi, Paola Di Stefano, Maria del Pilar Camacho Leal, Agata Tinnirello, Brigitte Bisaro, Virginia Morello, Laura Damiano, Simona Aramu, Daniele Repetto, Giusy Tornillo, and Paola Defilippi

Abstract 43
Overview of Integrin Structure 43
The SFK-Fak-p130Cas Signaling 46
Conclusion 52

6. PHYSICAL AND FUNCTIONAL INTERACTION BETWEEN INTEGRINS AND HERG1 CHANNELS IN CANCER CELLS 55

Serena Pillozzi and Annarosa Arcangeli

Abstract 55
Introduction 56
hERG1 Channels in Cancer Cells 56
Effects of Integrin Activation on hERG1 Channels 59
Integrins and hERG1 Channels form a Macromolecular Complex 61
Effects of hERG1 Activation on Integrin Function and Signaling 62
Conclusion 64

7. COORDINATED REGULATION OF VASCULAR CA^{2+} AND K$^+$ CHANNELS BY INTEGRIN SIGNALING 69

Peichun Gui, Jun-Tzu Chao, Xin Wu, Yan Yang, George E. Davis, and Michael J. Davis

Abstract 69
Introduction 69

Contents

Regulation of L-Type Calcium Channels by Integrin Activation 70
Regulation of Ca^{2+}-Dependent Potassium Channels by Integrin Activation 73
Conclusion 76

8. ADHESION-DEPENDENT MODULATION OF MACROPHAGE K+ CHANNELS 81

Margaret Colden-Stanfield

Abstract 81
Introduction 81
Inwardly Rectifying K+ (Kir) Currents 81
Physiologic and Pathophysiologic Roles of Macrophage Kir Channels 87
Delayed, Outwardly Rectifying K+ (Kdr) Currents 88
Physiologic and Pathophysiologic Roles of Macrophage Kdr Channels 89
Conclusion 92

9. INTEGRIN RECEPTORS AND LIGAND-GATED CHANNELS 95

Raffaella Morini and Andrea Becchetti

Abstract 95
Introduction 95
The Functional Significance of Integrins in the Adult Brain 96
Integrins and Nicotinic Acetylcholine Receptors:
    Not Only the Neuromuscular Junction 100
Conclusion 102

10. INTEGRINS AND ION CHANNELS IN CELL MIGRATION: IMPLICATIONS FOR NEURONAL DEVELOPMENT, WOUND HEALING AND METASTATIC SPREAD 107

Andrea Becchetti and Annarosa Arcangeli

Abstract 107
Introduction 108
The Role of Integrins in Cell Migration 110
The Role of Ion Channels and Crosstalk with Integrins in Cell Migration 111
Ca^{2+} Signaling and the Axonal Growth Cone 113
Ion Channels as Adhesion Molecules 115
The Cellular Environment and the Metastatic Process 115
Invasiveness of Glial Tumors and Ion Channels 118
Conclusion 118

INDEX 125

ACKNOWLEDGEMENTS

This work has been supported by the Italian Ministry of University and Scientific and Technological Research, the Italian Association for Cancer Research (AIRC), the Association for International Cancer Research (AICR), the Associazione Genitori Noi per Voi, the Ente Cassa di Risparmio di Firenze and the University of Milano-Bicocca, and the Istituto Toscano Tumori.

The editors wish to thank Professor Massimo Olivotto and Professor Enzo Wanke for advice and encouragement.

CHAPTER 1

Integrin Structure and Functional Relation with Ion Channels

Annarosa Arcangeli and Andrea Becchetti*

Abstract

Physical and functional link between cell adhesion molecules and ion channels provide a rapid connection between extracellular environment and cell physiology. Growing evidence does shows that frequent cross talk occurs between these classes of membrane proteins. These interactions are being addressed in ever increasing molecular detail. Recent advances have given X-ray resolved structure of the extracellular domains of integrin receptors. Such a level of resolution is still not available for the transmembrane and intracellular domains. Nonetheless, current molecular biological work is unraveling an intricate network connecting the cytoplasmic integrin domains with the cytoskeleton, ion channels and variety of cellular messengers. Overall, these studies show that integrins and ion channels both present bidirectional signaling features. Extracellular signals are usually transduced by integrins to trigger cellular responses that may involve ion fluxes, which can offer further relay. Intracellular processes and ion channel engagement can in turn affect integrin activation and expression and thus cell adhesion to the extracellular matrix. Moreover, ion channels themselves can communicate extracellular messages to both the cytoplasmic environment and integrin themselves. These interactions appear to often depend on formation of multiprotein membrane complexes that can recruit other elements, such as growth factor receptors and cytoplasmic signaling proteins. This chapter provides a general introduction to the field by giving a brief historical introduction and summarizing the main features of integrin structure and link to the cytoplasmic proteins. In addition, it outlines the main cellular processes in which channel-integrin interplay is known to exert clear physiological and pathological roles.

Introduction

Transmembrane ion fluxes through channels and transporters control a wide variety of cellular processes. Besides classic roles in regulating the action potential firing, synaptic transmission, cell motility and exocytosis, work carried out in the last two decades points to widespread implications in modulating the cellular state on a longer time scale. In addition, the asymmetrical arrangement of ion transport proteins typically found in the apical and basolateral membranes of epithelial layers, besides the obvious role in transepithelial transport, immediately suggests how tissues could produce steady currents at a supracellular level. This functional polarization is thought to contribute to the establishment of embryonal axes, organogenesis and wound healing.[1] As a consequence, ion channel malfunction can lead to a variety of serious diseases.

Most of the cellular activities outlined above strictly depend on extracellular context, whose nature is communicated to the intracellular environment by an array of integral membrane proteins that mediate cell adhesion to neighbouring cells and to the extracellular matrix (ECM).[2,3] Modern

*Corresponding Author: Andrea Becchetti—Department of Biotechnology and Biosciences, University of Milano-Bicocca, Piazza della Scienza 2, 20126 Milan, Italy. Email: andrea.becchetti@unimib.it

Integrins and Ion Channels: Molecular Complexes and Signaling, edited by Andrea Becchetti and Annarosa Arcangeli. ©2010 Landes Bioscience and Springer Science+Business Media.

biomolecular and cell physiological methods have led to an explosive growth of knowledge about the asymmetries at the molecular level that explain so much of the biological functional organization and that were largely unfathomable just a few decades ago (e.g., ref. 4).

Cell adhesion to the ECM is mostly mediated by integrin receptors, which are transmembrane proteins formed by noncovalently associated α and β subunits. Each subunit is a type I transmembrane glycoprotein with a relatively large multidomain extracellular portion, a single membrane spanning helix and a short (20 to 70 aminoacids), largely unstructured, cytoplasmic tail.[5] An exception is β4 subunit, which has a large (about 1000 amino acids) cytoplasmic domain.[6] Mammals contain 18 α and 8 β subunits that combine to produce at least 24 different heterodimers, each of which can bind to a specific repertoire of extracellular ligands such as fibronectin, collagen, laminin, or fibrinogen, or to cell surface counter-receptors like ICAM-1 or VCAM-1. Binding to ECM is regulated by conformational changes in the integrin extracellular domains driven by interaction of the cytoplasmic domain with cytoskeletal and signaling proteins.[7] In turn, cell adhesion recruits an array of cytoskeletal, scaffolding and signaling proteins that associate on integrin cytoplasmic face, giving rise to specific macromolecular structures called Focal Adhesions (FAs).[8] Hence, a bidirectional transmission of mechanical force and biochemical signals across the plasma membrane takes place through integrins. The ECM-dependent signals are transduced into cellular responses such as cell spreading, migration, proliferation and death ('outside-in' signaling), whereas integrin affinity for ECM and surface expression are in turn modulated by intracellular signals that thus control cell adhesion ('inside-out' signaling or integrin activation).[9,10]

While the importance of integrins in cell biology has been long recognized (for review of early literature, see ref. 3), detailed studies on how integrin-mediated adhesion affects cell signaling lagged considerably behind those carried out on neurotransmission or the cell's response to growth factors. Some degree of incommunicability between researchers in different fields perhaps contributed to such a delay, although the main reason was probably the sheer difficulty of carrying out physiological and biochemical experiments on adherent cells. For example, collecting cells for biochemical essays requires cell detachment from substrate, which unavoidably alters or interrupts the signal being studied. Another drawback is that signal kinetics is difficult to determine in cell adhesion processes, because it is impossible to apply and remove the stimulus at will, unless some soluble compound is available to mimic the effects of an ECM ligand. Only towards 1990, the cell physiological and the biomolecular methods reached a state of maturity sufficient to circumvent most of these experimental problems. In particular, the progressive development of patch-clamp methods and the production of intracellular probes for measuring ion activity with optical techniques gave better opportunities to study cell signaling in single mammalian adherent cells. The first such studies appeared in the early nineties, showing that integrin-mediated cell adhesion stimulates K^+ channel activity[11-13] and controls cell pH[14] and cytosolic free Ca^{2+}.[15] All of these effects have regulatory meaning for cell growth and differentiation. In parallel, similar methods were applied to the study of the regulatory interaction between cell-cell adhesion molecules and voltage-gated Ca^{2+} channels.[16]

Fundamentals of Integrin Structure

Extracellular Domains and ECM Ligand Binding

X-ray crystallography and NMR studies have recently offered great insight on the three-dimensional structure of the extracellular portion of integrin receptors. In general, two big classes of integrins are distinguished, depending on whether or not an extracellular von Willebrand factor type A domain is present in their α subunit. This domain is thus called αA or αI and is homologous to a typical GTPase domains, in which however the catalytic site is substituted with a metal ion-dependent adhesion site (MIDAS). MIDAS is normally occupied by a divalent cation enabling αA to modulate the divalent cation-dependence of ECM protein binding.[17] A full description of the complex conformational changes occurring on ligand binding is outside the scope of this review (for full treatment, see refs. 18-19). In brief, αA can assume either a low affinity ('closed') conformation or a high affinity ('open') conformation. The transition to the open state rearranges MIDAS so as to allow binding of an acidic residue on the ECM ligand. This residue thus offers the sixth coordination site for the divalent cation, substituting a water molecule present in the closed state.

The three-dimensional structure of the external domain of the integrins that lack αA was determined on the αVβ3 type.[20-22] AlphaV contains four domains: an N-terminal 'β-propeller', a 'Thigh' (Ig-like) domain, Calf-1 and Calf-2 (two β-sandwich domains). The β subunit contains instead eight domains: an N-terminal PSI (Plexin-Semaphorin-Integrin) followed by four EGF-like domains and a tail domain (βTD) close to the plasma membrane; the PSI domain wraps an Ig-like 'Hybrid' domain that contains, between its two β-sheets, the βA domain (structurally similar to αA).

Association of the propeller and the βA domains forms a 'head', which is thought to account for the formation of the αβ complex. Such a head resides onto 'legs' formed by the Thigh and Calf domains of αV and the PSI, Hybrid, EGFs and βTD domains of β3. The legs of the two integrin subunits interact at various points and are bent at 'knees' located between Hybrid and Calf-1 (in αV) and between EGF1 and EGF2 (in β3). The MIDAS of βA is not occupied by a metal cation, but a Ca^{2+} ion is typically located in an adjacent site (named ADMIDAS) that stabilizes the unliganded state. On the other hand, four metal ions bind the propeller domain of αV and a fifth binds Calf-1. The structure of the domains bound to ligands is usually studied by applying peptides containing the Arg-Gly-Asp (RGD) sequence. RGD is typically present in the ECM proteins that associate with integrins and mediates such an interaction. It turned out to insert between the propeller and βA domains. The D residue, in particular, binds a MIDAS occupied by a metal ion, similarly to the situation of αA.

The general interpretation of these and other structural data in terms of transmembrane signal transduction is still debated. A 'switchblade' activation model has been proposed for both types of integrin receptors, with the high-affinity state presenting an extension of the normally bent extracellular structure that allows integrin activation.[23] In alternative, a 'deadbolt' model proposes that relatively modest quaternary conformational rearrangements can account for integrin activation, being sufficient to conformational restructuring, especially of the F/α7 loop.[24]

Transmembrane and Intracellular Domains

The celebrated crystal structure that we have illustrated above does however not contain informations about the transmembrane (TM) and cytoplasmic domains, which we hereafter briefly survey. An extensive set of conclusive experiments has established the relevance of the TM domains of both α and β subunits for bidirectional signal transduction across the plasma membrane (reviewed in ref. 25). We will discuss the evidence for interaction between the TM regions of α and β subunits, as well as how 'inside-out' activation by proteins such as talin affects this interaction. Finally, we will examine the role of the β cytoplasmic domains for protein-protein interactions and for the link to the intracellular signalling machinery.

TM Domain Interaction

Across family members and species, the TM helices have a conserved but unusual pattern of hydrophobicity. Single-pass TM segments are thought to traverse the membrane as α-helices. In β subunits, helices contain a stretch of 23 mostly hydrophobic residues that terminates on the intracellular side with a Trp-Lys pair, or a similar residue combination. This is followed by another prevalently apolar stretch of residues that forms a substantial helix tilt relative to the membrane plane. Studies carried out on β3 integrins suggest that the helix tilt allows Lys 716 to 'snorkel' its side chain out of the hydrophobic lipid core.[26] The TM helices of the α subunits exhibit a similar pattern of hydrophobicity, except that they probably lack a significant helix tilt, as has been proven for αIIb.[27] The interaction between the α and β TM domains has been directly viewed with cryomicroscopy and single particle reconstruction of detergent-solubilised αIIb/β3 integrins. Additional evidence for inter-subunit interaction of the TM domains has come from cysteine-scanning mutagenesis experiments on αIIb/β3 integrin.[28] These experiments were consistent with a model in which the TM domains are bonded when inactive and separate in the active state, becoming capable of binding soluble ligands. Interestingly, 'outside-in' activation does not appear to require the separation of the TM domains, while 'inside-out' activation does. Förster Resonance Energy Transfer (FRET)[29] studies on intact αLβ2 integrins not only agree with the idea that TM segments separate on activation, but indicate that this also applies to the cytoplasmic domains. FRET experiments also confirm that tail separation is not required for 'outside-in' activation.

Several models have been proposed to explain how conformational changes in the cytoplasmic tails affect the conformation of the ectodomain. These generally consider the occurrence of changes in the position of the TM domains within the bilayer, which in turn cause the extracellular domains to move to the active state. Once again, a full description of these models is beyond our purposes. In brief, the one that has gained wider consent is probably the TM domain "separation" model. At rest, the inactive receptor state is stabilized by hydrophobic packing of the TM helices and by electrostatic interactions between the adjacent α and β subunits. Integrin activation ensues from movement and complete separation of the TM segments.[25]

Inside-Out Activation by Talin

How does integrin activation occur? Although the precise structural and topological processes underlying this mechanism are still debated, the 'inside-out' activation process is generally thought to require interaction between cytoplasmic ligands and the integrin tails. In this way, a conformational change is triggered that is transmitted to the extracellular ligand-binding domains through the TM and stalk regions. One such ligand is the cytoplasmic protein talin. Talin consists of a ~50 kDa head region and a ~200 kDa rod segment. Head contains a 300-residue FERM (protein 4.1, ezrin, rodixin, moesin) domain, composed by F1, F2 and F3 subdomains. Rod consists of a series of α-helical bundles. Talin can bind both to the integrin cytoplasmic domains and to vinculin and actin filaments, thus connecting the cytoskeleton and the ECM. In particular, the FERM domain has binding sites for the cytoplasmic domain of β-integrins and laylin (a hyaluronan receptor) as well as for filamentous actin (F-actin). The tail head also binds to two signaling molecules that regulate the dynamics of FAs, namely the focal adhesion kinase (FAK) and the phosphatidylinositol (4)-phosphate-5-kinase type Iγ (PIPKIγ90). Intact talin is relatively ineffectual at activating integrins and needs stimulation to trigger significant activation. This implies that their integrin binding sites are masked, in the intact molecule. Cleavage between the head and rod domains by the protease calpain, for example, results in a 16-fold increase in binding to β3 integrin tails. A similar effect is produced by PIP2 binding to talin. Integrin activation is mediated by the head domain. In particular, the F3 subdomain of FERM contains a phosphotyrosine binding domain (PTB) that binds the more N-terminal of the two NPxY motifs found in the cytoplasmic domains of β-integrins. The NPxY sequences are typical targets for PTB domains, but several other PTB-containing proteins can bind to the same motif without producing integrin activation. Therefore, talin's F3 must make additional contacts with the integrin cytoplasmic domain. The current model is that talin initiates integrin activation by disrupting a salt bridge between the α and β integrin subunits, which disrupts their interface and leads to separation of their cytoplasmic domains. Such a model is supported by FRET studies on αLβ2 integrins.[25]

The talin-mediated integrin activation is stimulated by intracellular messengers such as the small GTPase Rap1A. The latter is in turn regulated by protein kinase C, as shown by reconstituting platelet integrin αIIb/β3 activation in CHO cells. A further mediator of talin activation is the Rap1A-interacting adaptor molecule (RIAM), but other mechanisms for regulating talin and its association with integrins have been suggested.[30] As to the outside-in pathways, integrin signaling via FAK and Src promotes binding of PIPK1γ90 to the talin's F3 domain, with ensuing activation of PIPKγ90 and translocation of complex to the plasma membrane. Hence, current evidence suggests that a self-sustaining mechanism depending on integrin-mediated signaling maintains integrin activation.

To make the picture more complex, the talin's rod contains an additional integrin-binding site, at least two actin-binding sites and several binding sites for vinculin, which itself has multiple partners. The talin's rod binds to a hydrophobic pocket in the vinculin head through 10 of its 62 amphipathic α-helices. Conversely, binding to F-actin depends on talin dimerization, which occurs through the monomer's C-terminal helices.

Binding to Other Membrane Proteins and Cytoskeleton

Integrins are typically linked to the actin cytoskeleton, with the exception of α5β4, usually coupled to intermediate filaments. As detailed above, talin plays a pivotal role in connecting most integrin types to F-actin filaments. However, both β and α cytoplasmic tails are known to bind to many other proteins, with consequent mechanical and signaling effects. Formation of FAs is particularly dependent on these tails.[31] An example is the interaction of α4 with paxillin, although link to β-tails is much more common. To date, more than 70 intracellular proteins have been reported to bind integrin tails, with variable specificities. Partners include α-actinin, filamin, tensin, integrin-linked-kinase, melusin and skelemin.[25,31]

It is possible that the β-tail's availability to form a "hub" for a large number of proteins depends on its intrinsic disordered structure.[32] In fact, despite of its shortness, the β-tail can extend over a significant distance (8 nm) because of this property. Moreover, the β-tail provides multiple protein binding sites. For example, it usually contains several NPxY sequences. Therefore, as a working hypothesis, it is often sensible to suppose that the integrin β-tail is the domain involved in the interaction with ion channel proteins.[33]

Physiological and Pathological Implications: An Outline of Current Trends

Consistent with integrin association with the cytoskeleton, the cell adhesion machinery often transduces mechanical strain into modification of ion fluxes. A typical response is increase of free $[Ca^{2+}]_i$, as is testified by work in endothelium, fibroblasts and vascular smooth muscle. These responses often involve tyrosine kinase cascades.[34,35] The relevance for vascular control is fully discussed in Chapter 7. We add here that modulation of Ca^{2+} homeostasis is certainly not the only effect of mechanical signals. In ventricular myocytes in particular, β1 integrin stretch leads to activation of swell-activated Cl⁻ currents, under control of (i) tyrosine kinase-dependent signaling (centered on Src and FAK) and (ii) the pathway that converges on reactive oxygen species (centered on phosphatidyl inositol-3 kinase and NADPH oxidase). Because this pathway is also activated by the angiotensin II receptor AT1, it is likely that the interplay of these pathways is involved in the frequent activation of the swell-activated Cl⁻ channels in different models of cardiac disease.[36-38]

Integrin engagement is also relevant for immune cell response. An example are human T-cells, which highlight some further typical features of the integrin-channel cross-talk. Biochemical evidence suggests that $K_v1.3$ voltage-gated K^+ channels activate integrin function through formation of a membrane complex. In addition, T-cells also express ionotropic glutamate receptors and both K^+ fluxes and extracellular glutamate can activate integrin-mediated adhesion.[39,40] This shows that reciprocal signaling is common: cell adhesion to the extracellular matrix can induce channel activation and, in turn, channel engagement can lead to regulate cell adhesion. Therefore, the bidirectional nature of integrin-mediated signaling is also presented by ion channels themselves, that both respond to and regulate cell adhesion. Moreover, these mechanisms can depend on formation of multiprotein membrane complexes.

Another piece of the jigsaw is contributed by studies pointing to a channel-mediated regulation of integrin expression. The first evidence about channel control of integrin expression was obtained in the preosteoclastic leukemia cell line FLG 29.1. Activation of the *ether-à-go-go* related type 1 K^+ channels (hERG1) during β1 integrin-mediated cell adhesion stimulates surface expression of αVβ3 integrins. Hence the signals centered on the ion channel constitute a regulatory network that connects different integrin subunits.[41] Evidences along similar lines have been obtained for glutamate receptors. Aside from typical integrin-mediated control through phosphorylation cascades (on NMDA receptors),[42,43] it turns out that AMPA receptor activation stimulates membrane expression of α5β1 integrins.[44] The implications for neuronal plasticity and development are fully discussed in Chapter 9.

Conclusion

Finally, the results on leukemic cell lines brings us to comment about the relevance of the above studies for oncology, another rapidly growing field. The implications for neoplastic progression are immediately suggested by the many evidences showing that the integrin-channel interplay controls cell adhesion, differentiation and migration. Blood cells offer particularly favourable experimental conditions and are being intensely studied from this standpoint. For example, in acute myeloid leukemia, hERG1 channels and β1 integrins physically associate with the vascular endothelial growth factor receptor 1. Recent data in vitro and in vivo show that hERG1 mediates the growth factor-dependent cell migration and invasion, thus enhancing malignancy.[45] These studies are fully discussed in Chapter 6.

References

1. McCaig CD, Rajnicek AM, Song B et al. Controlling cell behavior electrically: current views and future potential. Physiol Rev 2005; 85:943-978.
2. Edelman GM. Cell adhesion molecules in the regulation of animal form and tissue pattern. Annu Rev Cell Biol 1986; 2:81-116.
3. Hynes RO. Integrins: versatility, modulation and signaling in cell adhesion. Cell 1992; 69:11-25.
4. Needham J. Order and life. Yale University Press, 1936.
5. Hynes RO. Integrins: Bidirectional, allosteric signalling machines. Cell 2002; 110:673-687.
6. dePereda JM, Wiche G, Liddington RC. Crystal structure of a tandem pair of fibronectin type III domains from the cytoplasmic tail of integrin α6β4. EMBO J 1999; 18:4087-4095.
7. Liddington RC, Ginsberg MH. Integrin activation takes shape. J Cell Biol 2002; 158:833-839.
8. Miranti CK, Brugge JS. Sensing the environment. A historical perspective of integrin signal transduction. Nat Cell Biol 2002; 4:E83-E90.
9. Schwartz MA. Integrin signaling revisited. Trends Cell Biol 2001; 11:466-470.
10. Ginsberg MH, Partridge A, Shattil SJ. Integrin regulation. Curr Opin Cell Biol 2005; 17:509-516.
11. Arcangeli A, Becchetti A, Del Bene MR et al. Fibronectin-integrin binding promotes hyperpolarization of murine erythroleukemia cells. Biochem Biophys Res Commun 1991; 177:1266-1272.
12. Becchetti A, Arcangeli A, Del Bene MR et al. Response to fibronectin-integrin interaction in leukaemia cells: delayed enhancing of a K$^+$ current. Proc Roy Soc Lond B 1992; 248:235-240.
13. Arcangeli A, Becchetti A, Mannini A et al. Integrin-mediated neurite outgrowth in neuroblastoma cells depends on the activation of potassium channels. J Cell Biol 1993; 122:1131-1143.
14. Ingber DE, Prusty D, Frangioni JV et al. Control of intracellular pH and growth by fibronectin in capillary endothelial cells. J Cell Biol 1990; 110:1803-1811.
15. Jaconi MEE, Theler JM, Schlegel W et al. Multiple elevations of cytosolic free Ca^{2+} in human neutrophils: initiation by adherence receptors of the integrin family. J Cell Biol 1991; 112:1249-1257.
16. Doherty P, Ashton SV, Moore SE et al. Morphoregulatory activities of NCAM and N-cadherin can be accounted for by G-protein dependent activation of L- and N-type neuronal calcium channels. Cell 1991; 67:21-33.
17. Michishita M, Videm V, Arnaout MA. A novel divalent cation-binding site in the A domain of the beta 2 integrin CR3 (CD11b/CD18) is essential for ligand binding. Cell 1993; 72:857-867.
18. Arnaout MA, Goodman SL, Xiong JP. Structure and mechanics of integrin-based cell adhesion. Curr Opin Cell Biol 2007; 19:495-507.
19. Arnaout MA, Mahalingam B, Xiong JP. Integrin structure, allostery and bidirectional signaling. Annu Rev Cell Dev Biol 2005; 21:381-410.
20. Xiong JP, Stehle T, Diefenbach B et al. Crystal structure of the extracellular segment of integrin alphaVbeta3. Science 2001; 294:339-345.
21. Xiong JP, Stehle T, Zhang R et al. Crystal structure of the extracellular segment of integrin alphaVbeta3 in complex with an Arg-Gly-Asp ligand. Science 2002; 296:151-155.
22. Xiong JP, Stehle T, Goodman SL et al. A novel adaptation of the integrin PSI domain revealed from its crystal structure. J Biol Chem 2004; 279:40252-40254.
23. Nishida N, Xie C, Shimaoka M et al. Activation of leukocyte beta(2) integrins by conversion from bent to extended conformation. Immunity 2006; 25:583-594.
24. Xiong JP, Stehle T, Goodman SL et al. New insights into the structural basis of integrin activation. Blood 2003; 102:1155-1159.
25. Wegener KL, Campbell ID. Transmembrane and cytoplasmic domains in integrin activation and protein-protein interactions. Mol Membr Biol 2008; 25:376-387.
26. Lau TL, Partridge AW, Ginsberg MH et al. Structure of the integrin β3 transmembrane segment in phospholipid bicelles and detergent micelles. Biochemistry 2008; 47:4008-4016.

27. Lau T-L, Dua V, Ulmer TS. Structure of the integrin αIIb transmembrane segment. J Biol Chem 2008; 283:16162-16168.
28. Luo BH, Springer TA, Takagi J. A specific interface between integrin transmembrane helices and affinity for ligand. PLoS Biol 2004; 2:776-786.
29. Kim M, Carman CV, Springer TA. Bidirectional transmembrane signaling by cytoplasmic domain separation in integrins. Science 2003; 301:1720-1725.
30. Critchley DR, Gingras AR. Talin at a glance. J Cell Sci 2008; 121:1345-1347.
31. Critchley DR. Focal adhesions—the cytoskeletal connections. Curr Opin Cell Biol 2000; 12:133-139.
32. Dunker AK, Cortese MS, Romero P et al. Flexible nets. The roles of intrinsic disorder in protein interaction networks. FEBS J 2005; 272:5129-5148.
33. Cherubini A, Hofmann G, Pillozzi S et al. Human ether-à-go-go-related gene 1 channels are physically linked to beta1 integrins and modulate adhesion-dependent signaling. Mol Biol Cell 2005; 16:2972-2983.
34. Davis MJ. Regulation of ion channels by integrins. Cell Biochem Biophys 2002; 36:41-66.
35. Arcangeli A, Becchetti A. Complex functional interaction between integrin receptors and ion channels. Trends Cell Biol 2006; 16:632-639.
36. Browe DM, Baumgarten CM. Stretch of beta 1 integrin activates an outwardly rectifying chloride current via FAK and Src in rabbit ventricular myocytes. J Gen Physiol 2003; 122:689-702.
37. Browe DM, Baumgarten CM. EGFR kinase regulates volume-sensitive chloride current elicited by integrin stretch via PI-3K and NADPH oxidase in ventricular myocytes. J Gen Physiol 2006; 127:237-251.
38. Ren Z, Raucci FJ, Browe DM et al. Regulation of swelling-activated Cl⁻ currents by angiotensin II signalling and NADPH oxidase in rabbit ventricle. Cardiovasc Res 2008; 77:73-80.
39. Levite M, Cahalon L, Peretz A et al. Extracellular K⁺ and opening of voltage-gated potassium channels activate T-cell integrin function: physical and functional association between Kv1.3 channels and beta1 integrins. J Exp Med 2001; 191:1167-1176.
40. Ganor Y, Besser M, Ben-Zakay N et al. Human T-cells express a functional ionotropic glutamate receptor GluR3 and glutamate by itself triggers integrin-mediated adhesion to laminin and fibronectin and chemotactic migration. J Immunol 2003; 170:4362-4372.
41. Hofmann G, Bernabei PA, Crociani O et al. hERG K⁺ channels activation during β_1 integrin-mediated adhesion to fibronectin induces an up regulation of $\alpha_V\beta_3$ integrin in the preosteoclastic leukemia cell line FLG 29.1. J Biol Chem 2001; 276:4923-4931.
42. Lin B, Arai AC, Lynch G et al. Integrins regulate NMDA receptor-mediated synaptic currents. J Neurophysiol 2003; 89:2874-2878.
43. Bernard-Trifilo JA, Kramar AE, Torp R et al. Integrin signaling cascades are operational in adult hippocampal synapses and modulate NMDA receptor physiology. J Neurochem 2005; 93:834-849.
44. Lin C-Y, Lynch G, Gall, CM. AMPA receptor stimulation increases alpha5beta1 integrin surface expression, adhesive function and signaling. J Neurochem 2005; 94:531-546.
45. Pillozzi S, Brizzi MF, Bernabei PA et al. VEGFR-1 (FLT-1), β_1 integrin and hERG K⁺ channel form a macromolecular signaling complex in acute myeloid leukemia: role in cell migration and clinical outcome. Blood 2007; 110:1238-1250.

CHAPTER 2

Introduction to Ion Channels

Chiara Di Resta and Andrea Becchetti*

Abstract

Ion channels are integral membrane proteins that contain pathways through which ions can flow. By shifting between closed and open conformational states ('gating' process), they control passive ion flow through the plasma membrane. Channels can be gated by membrane potential, or specific ligands, or other agents, such as mechanical stimuli. The efficacy of the gating process and the kinetics of subsequent inactivation or desensitization are regulated by intracellular mechanisms. Many types of membrane channels exist, with different degrees of ion selectivity. By controlling ion fluxes, they typically regulate membrane potential and excitability, shape the action potential, trigger muscle contraction and exocytosis (through Ca^{2+} influx), regulate cell volume and many other cellular processes. In the first part of the chapter, we give a brief introduction to the main physiological aspects of ion channels, which may not be familiar to molecular biologists. Subsequently, as a reference for later chapters, we summarize the main structural and functional features of the channel-proteins presently known to be related to integrin receptors.

Introduction

The fundamentals of cell physiology were established before 1970. Among the major achievements, we recall the determination of the ionic basis of action potential by A.L. Hodgkin and A.F. Huxley in the fifties, the discovery of the Na^+ pump by J.C. Skou (1957) and the elucidation of the fundamental synaptic mechanisms by S. Kuffler, B. Katz, R. Miledi, J.C. Eccles and others, in the fifties and sixties.[1-4]

Although many researchers had long thought that transmembrane ion fluxes depended on conduction pathways located within specific membrane proteins,[5] this could only be demonstrated around 1980, with the progressive convergence of ever more sophisticated biophysical and molecular biological methods. A story of these seminal studies, mostly focused on synaptic mechanisms, is found in ref. 6. The first ion channel to be isolated both biophysically and biochemically was the muscular acetylcholine receptor (also called nicotinic receptor, nAChR, because it and its neuronal homologues can be activated by nicotine). In the mid-seventies, several groups were attempting to purify the nAChR's subunits from the electroplaques of *Torpedo*, an electric fish in which it is densely expressed.[6] The first cloning of the α subunit came out from S. Numa's laboratory in 1982.[7] However, detailed structural information lagged behind because of the difficulties encountered in crystallizing membrane proteins. The first X-ray resolved structure of an ion channel was actually obtained much later, for a voltage-gated K^+ channel obtained from the bacterium *Streptomyces lividans*.[8] This study primed a fruitful course of research that is now leading to high-resolution structural maps of other membrane channels (e.g., ref. 9).

From a functional point of view, the first registration of a current flowing through a single channel was reported in 1976 by E. Neher and B. Sakmann, who deviced the patch-clamp method and applied

*Corresponding author: Andrea Becchetti—Department of Biotechnology and Biosciences, University of Milano-Bicocca. Piazza della Scienza, 2. 20126 Milano, Italy. Email: andrea.becchetti@unimib.it

Integrins and Ion Channels: Molecular Complexes and Signaling, edited by Andrea Becchetti and Annarosa Arcangeli. ©2010 Landes Bioscience and Springer Science+Business Media.

it to nAChRs on denervated muscle.[10,11] With this technique, a very tight seal is established between a glass pipette's rim and the plasma membrane, thus isolating small membrane patch. The ensuing decrease in background electrical noise allows one to reliably measure currents of the order of pA, the typical magnitude of unitary currents. If the membrane patch is gently ruptured, electrical access is obtained to the currents flowing through the entire cell's membrane. This technique permits to study cells of any size, because patch-clamp pipettes are much less invasive than classical microelectrodes. Therefore, the last twenty-five years have witnessed an explosive growth of mammalian cell physiology. This has led not only to more detailed understanding of excitability, but also to reveal ion channel implications in many other cellular processes such as cell cycle, substrate adhesion, motility, etc.

The Physiology of Ion Channels

Accessible introductions to electrodiffusion through biological membranes are found in refs. 12-13. More advanced treatments are found in refs. 14-15. By convention, the membrane electric potential (or membrane voltage, V_m) is the difference between the intracellular and the extracellular V. Hence, when V_m equals −80 mV, say, the internal side of the membrane is 80 mV more negative than the extracellular side.

Biophysical Background

Ion channels are integral membrane proteins, composed of different subunits or domains that usually surround a central pore, although channels containing multiple pores are also known. Typically, the conductive pathway is 'gated' by a conformational transition energetically driven by V_m (voltage-gated channels) or ligand binding (ligand-gated channels). This process (activation) can also be driven by other mechanisms, such as membrane stretch (mechanically-gated channels). The probability of channel opening in the presence of the activating factor can be regulated, e.g., by phosphorylation or allosteric modulation. If the stimulus is removed, channels close (deactivation). The deactivated state is the closed state typical of resting condition. On the other hand, if the activating factor persists, most channel types progressively tend to reach a closed state different from the deactivated state, by a process called inactivation (for voltage-gated channels) or desensitization. The kinetics of inactivation/desensitization ranges from milliseconds to minutes, depending on channel type and conditions. If the stimulus is removed after inactivation or desensitization has taken place, the channel cannot be immediately reactivated by further stimulus application, but a certain time is required for the protein to come back to the resting closed state, which is available for activation. Once again, the kinetics of such a recovery is variable. An example of activation, desensitization and deactivation is shown in Figure 1A, for a ligand-gated channel (a neuronal nAChR) treated with nicotine.

A central concept in cell physiology is the equilibrium (or Nernst) potential for a certain ion i (E_i). E_i is the V_m value at which the i's membrane net flow caused by the trasmembrane concentration gradient is balanced by the flow in the opposite direction driven by the transmembrane electric field. Thus, when $V_m = E_i$, the net current for i is null. E_i depends on the transmembrane concentration gradients established for i by the active transporters, such as the Na$^+$/K$^+$ ATPase and the Ca$^+$ ATPase. It can be calculated by using the Nernst equation:

$$E_i = \frac{RT}{zF} \ln \frac{[i]_o}{[i]_{in}}$$

where R is the gas constant, T is the absolute temperature, z is i's valence, F is the Faraday constant, $[i]_o$ and $[i]_{in}$ are i's concentrations in the extra- and intracellular medium, respectively. For example, at the typical extra- and intracellular concentrations of K$^+$ (in mammals) E_K is about −100 mV, at room temperature. Suppose a cell membrane only expresses K$^+$ channels (and these are perfectly selective). When they are open, K$^+$ tends on average to leave the cell because of the concentration gradient. However, K$^+$ efflux makes V_m increasingly more negative. At -100 mV, the efflux would be balanced by the influx caused by the electric field and the net transmembrane flux would be null. Were V_m more negative than E_K, the electric field would take over the effect produced by the concentration gradient and the net K$^+$ flux would be inward.

The above discussion is simplified in that no ion channel is perfectly selective. Strictly speaking, the V_m at which the net current flowing through a certain channel type is zero is named reversal potential (V_{rev}). When an ion channel is very selective for the ion i, it is a good approximation to assume that $V_{rev} \sim E_i$. Otherwise, V_{rev} depends on the pore permeability for different ions, among those present at significant levels in the extra- and intracellular solutions. For example, if a certain channel is permeable to Na$^+$ and K$^+$, V_{rev} will be located between E_K and E_{Na}, with the precise value depending on the relative permeabilities for these ions. Such a channel, poorly discriminating between Na$^+$ and K$^+$, will be probably also permeable to other alkali cations (such as Li$^+$, Rb$^+$, etc.), but these can be usually discounted, since their concentration in physiological solutions is negligible.

By analogy to Ohm's law, the current flowing through an ensemble of similar channels expressed within a certain membrane area can be expressed as:

$$I_r = G_r(V_m - V_{rev})$$

where I_r is the total current flowing through the channel Type r and G_r is the total conductance (i.e., the reciprocal of resistance R_r) for these channels. The (V_m-V_{rev}) factor is often called driving force. In general, G_r is not a constant. It is the product of the single-channel conductance (γ_r, which depends, among other things, on the interaction between the flowing ions and the conduction pathway), the number of channels r expressed onto the plasma membrane (N_r) and the probability that an individual channel be open (P_o). P_o usually depends on time (because of desensitization, say), on activating factors (such as V_m or agonist concentration) and many other factors (regulatory compounds, etc.). Thus:

$$I_r = \gamma_r N_r P_o(V,t,...)(V_m - E_{rev})$$

Main Physiological Roles of Ion Channels

A cell's V_m depends on which and how many channels are open at a given time. When K$^+$ channels predominate (as it is often the case in resting conditions, at least for excitable cells), V_m tends to E_K. When Na$^+$ channels predominate (e.g., at the action potential peak), V_m tends to E_{Na} (around +70 mV). The situation for Cl$^-$ is more complex, because the intracellular Cl$^-$ concentration is variable, depending not only on cell type (e.g., 30 mM in mammalian astrocytes and about 7 mM in neurons)[16] but also on the developmental stage. Developing neurons have usually higher [Cl$^-$]$_i$ than adult ones.[17] Ligand-gated channels are often poorly selective. For example, nicotinic receptors, glutamate receptors and cyclic nucleotide gated channels poorly discriminate between Na$^+$ and K$^+$ (the main physiological cations). Their V_{rev} is thus usually around the midpoint between E_K and E_{Na} (about −20/0 mV). When they are open, these channels tend to depolarize the membrane. In addition, they are often also permeable to Ca^{2+}, which has important implications for intracellular signaling. The classical physiological roles of voltage-gated channels are the shaping of action potentials in excitable cells (typically neurons, muscle cells and many sensory and endocrine cells). In addition, voltage-gated Ca^{2+} channels trigger muscle contraction and exocytosis. Ligand-gated channels typically control the synaptic function by making easier (excitation) or more difficult (inhibition) for a cell's to fire an action potential, in response to synaptic bombardment a certain transmitter. Other channel types control transepithelial ion flow, sensory transduction, etc.[12-15] Less conventional ion channel roles will be treated in other chapters.

Finally, a common term in biophysical jargon is rectification. It derives from electronics, where a rectifier is a circuit component that permits more current to flow in one direction than the other. An ion channel is said to present inward rectification if it conducts more easily currents flowing towards the cytoplasm, at a given driving force amplitude. When the opposite holds, the channel is an outward rectifier. For example, if E_K is −100 mV, a K$^+$ channel is called an inward rectifier if the current at (say) −140 mV (flowing inward because the driving force is −40 mV) is bigger than the current at −60 mV (flowing outward because the driving force is +40 mV). A certain degree of rectification is predicted by simple electrodiffusion, because current is bigger when ions flow from the more concentrated to the less concentrated side.[15] However, many channel types present

Integrin and Ion Channels: Molecular Complexes and Signaling

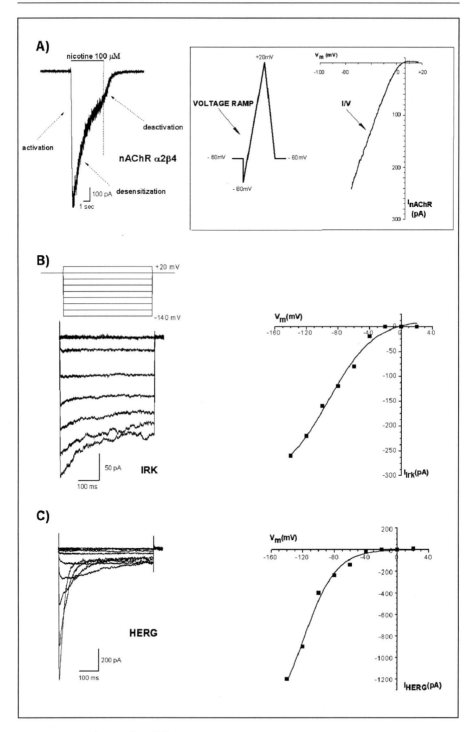

Figure 1. Legend viewed on following page.

Figure 1. Functional properties of some ion channels linked to integrins, studied in patch-clamp. A) Human neuronal heteromeric ($\alpha 2\beta 4$) nAChRs expressed in human embryonic kidney cells. Left panel: typical whole-cell current trace elicited by 100 μM nicotine, at –60 mV. Continuous bar marks time of agonist application. Arrows indicate the activation, desensitization and deactivation phases. Inset: current voltage (I/V) relation for neuronal nAChRs, measured by applying a 200 ms voltage ramp from –80 mV to +20 mV, as indicated. Holding V_m was –60 mV. Nicotinic current was elicited by 100 μM nicotine and isolated by subtracting the background current obtained in the absence of agonist. Notice the current rectification at V_m's more positive than V_{rev} (around –5 mV). Currents were recorded in the presence of physiological concentrations of the main ions, at room temperature. B) Inward rectifying K$^+$ channels from cultured astrocytes. Currents were elicited by applying voltage steps from –140 mV to +20 mV, as indicated. In these experiments, E_K was –30 mV, because the extracellular [K$^+$] was 40 mM. Notice that IRK currents are negligible at V_m more positive than V_{rev}. This is shown more clearly in the right panel, in which a current-voltage plot for IRK was obtained by plotting the peak currents as a function of test potential. IRK current was isolated by subtracting to the total current the backgroud currents measured in the presence of 100 μM Ba^{2+}, which strongly inhibits IRK channels. The slight time-dependent current decline at very negative V_m's is usually attributed to slow partial block by extracellular Na$^+$. C) Current voltage relation for HERG voltage-gated K$^+$ channels, spontaneosly expressed in human adenoma cells. Stimulation protocol and extracellular solutions were same as for IRK. Before applying the test V_m's, currents were activated/inactivated at 0 mV, for 10 s. When cells are brought to negative V_m, channel quickly deinactivate, revealing HERG current, whose amplitude increases as V_m gets farther from E_K (about –30 mV). Subsequently, channels deactivate, with a quicker kinetics, at more negative V_m's. HERG currents can be isolated from background by applying specific inhibitors, such as Way 123398 or E4031 (see Chapter 6). The right panel shows the corresponding I/V curve, measured from the peak currents shown in the left panel.

much more drastic rectification, because of voltage-dependent inhibition by intra- or extracellular compounds (as it is usually the case for ligand-gated channels or inward rectifying K$^+$ channels, Fig. 1A,B) or because of intrinsic voltage-dependence (e.g., Fig. 3C).

Ion Channel Types Involved in Integrin-Mediated Signaling

Voltage-Gated K$^+$ Channels

The voltage-gated K$^+$ channel families (K$_V$1 to K$_V$12) comprise different subtypes (named K$_V$1.1, K$_V$1.2, etc.).[18] A partial list is given in Table 1. They are composed of four identical α subunits, surrounding a central pore (Fig. 2). Each subunit contains an intracellular N-terminal domain, followed by six transmembrane domains (S1 to S6) and an intracellular C-terminal domain. The S4 domain is rich of basic aminoacid residues, whose side-chains are potentially positively charged and are thought to be responsible for the voltage-sensitivity. K$_V$ subunits are structurally related to the main subunits of the cyclic nucleotide-gated (CNG) channels. These are however largely insensitive to V_m and are instead gated by cyclic nucleotide binding to an intracellular nucleotide binding domain (NBD) located towards the C terminus. In fact, some K$_V$ channels (to be discussed later) do contain an intracellular segment highly homologous to NBD, which seems however to be non functional. The loop between S5 and S6 is named pore-loop (P-loop) or H5 domain. It lines the extracellular portion of the pore and determines not only ion selectivity but also gating, in both K$_V$ and CNG channels.[19-23] The α subunits can be modulated by a number of accessory subunits (Table 1).

Among the K$_V$ channels known to be related to integrin signaling, we recall that K$_V$1.3 is a delayed rectifying channel, i.e., it is activated (with a certain delay) by membrane depolarization. Therefore it only conducts net outward currents. In excitable cells, outwardly rectifying voltage-gated K$^+$ channels are typically activated by the depolarizing phase of the action potential and bring about cell's repolarization. These ion channels are also known to participate to a variety of other functions, from regulation of the G$_1$/S phase progression[24] to spatial buffering of K$^+$ by cerebral astrocytes in the brain.[25]

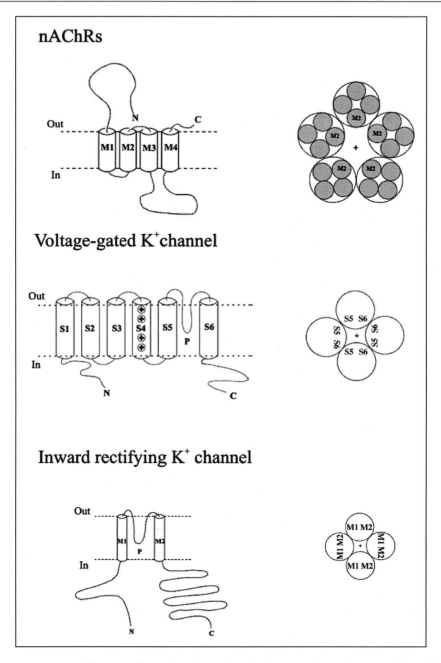

Figure 2. Structural features of some ligand-gated and voltage-gated ion channels. Left panels: Schematic structures of the typical subunit of nAChRs, voltage-gated K+ channels and inward rectifying K+ channels, as indicated. N and C indicate the N- and C- terminus, respectively. Dashed lines mark the plasma membrane borders. 'In' and 'out' mark the intra- and extracellular sides, respectively. Panels also indicate the transmembrane domains and the P loops (when present). Right panels illustrate the presumable subunit arrangement of the pentameric nAChRs and the tetrameric K+ channels.

Another family of voltage-gated channels related to integrins is K_V11 (also known as ERG, from *Ether-à-go-go* Related Gene, HERG in humans). K_V11 activates slowly on depolarizing from a negative V_m. Superimposed to activation, a quicker inactivation process takes place.[26] On first approximation, activation and inactivation can be assumed to be independent molecular processes. Thus, at a given V_m, the steady state current carried by a voltage-gated channel is proportional to the product of the probability that the channel is active (i.e., that the activating gate is open) times the probability that the channel is not inactive (i.e., that the inactivating gate is also in the open state). At the steady-state, little current is carried by ERG at V_m around 0 or positive, because the activating gate is open, but at the same time the inactivation domain blocks the channel. Inactivation is rapidly removed on cell repolarization. Therefore ERG currents can contribute significantly to the action potential repolarization, when both the activation and the inactivation gates are in a permissive position, for a brief time. Subsequently, at negative V_m, channels quickly deactivate (Fig. 1C). The physiological meaning of ERG kinetics has been extensively studied in cardiac myocytes,[27] much less in neurons (where this channel type is also widely expressed).[28] Particularly relevant for our purposes (see Chapter 6) are the steady state properties. All the ERG clones known to date generate appreciable stationary currents around −40 mV, a crucial V_m range for cycling cells. ERG gating and expression in fact oscillate during cell cycle (for review, see ref. 29). From a structural point of view, the *herg* gene (coding for HERG1) is formed by 15 exons, most coding for the N- and C- termini. The C-terminus contains a nonfunctional CNB domain. The N-terminus is formed by a terminal eag domain (1-135, in HERG1) and a proximal domain (136 to about 366). The former domain is a PAS (from the gene products of Per, Arnt and Sim) eukaryotic domain, homologous to similar domains present in Prokaryotes and involved in sensing environmental cues such as the redox state, light etc.[30] Both domains regulate channel function. Finally, at least two splicing forms of the murine and human ERG1 clones are known, ERG1a (full length clone) and ERG1b (N-terminal truncated form).[31] The latter tends to favour cell depolarization and is upregulated during S, in certain cell lines.[32]

Inward Rectifying K+ Channels

Inward rectifiers (Kir) preferentially conduct when V_m is more negative than E_K (Fig. 1B). This property mostly depends on voltage-dependent channel block by intracellular cations, particularly Mg^{2+} and the polyamines normally present in the cytoplasm (such as spermine and spermidine). The block is progressively more efficient at more positive V_m.[33] In this manner, Kir channels stabilize V_m around E_K in resting conditions, without short-circuiting the action potential when V_m depolarizes. This facilitates the production of action potentials with long plateaus in cardiac cells and oocytes, for example. Moreover, glial Kir participate to spatial buffering of K^+ in the brain. Kir subunits are coded by the *KCNJ1-KCNJ16* genes (Table 1). Differently from voltage-gated K^+ channels, they only present two transmembrane domains (M1 and M2, homologous to S5 and S6 of K_V channels), but retain a P-loop (Fig. 2).[34,35]

Ca2+-Activated K+ Channels

The subunits of the K^+ channels regulated by intracellular Ca^{2+} are collectively named K_{Ca}.[36-38] They are listed, with the corresponding genes, in Table 1. Traditionally, these channels were classified on the basis of single channel conductance. BK channels ($K_{Ca}1.1$) have particularly high γ (around 250 pS) and are activated by depolarization and $[Ca^{2+}]_i$, independently and synergistically. In $K_{Ca}1.1$, the typical module with S1-S6 transmembrane domains, homologous to that of K_V subunits, is preceded by a supplementary transmembrane segment (named S0). Voltage gating depends on a charged S4. The intracellular C-terminal domain is particularly elongated and contains regulatory sites sensitive to Ca^{2+} and other intracellular messengers. Similar structural features are presented by $K_{Ca}4.1$, $K_{Ca}4.2$ and $K_{Ca}5.1$. However, $K_{Ca}4$ channels are not voltage-dependent, because of S4 neutralization and appear to be activated by Na^+ instead of Ca^{2+} (at least in mammals). The other types of K_{Ca} known to date are named SK (small conductance, $K_{Ca}2$) and IK (intermediate conductance, $K_{Ca}3$) channels. These also retain the basic structure derived from K_V channels, but are not voltage-dependent, because of partial neutralization of the S4 residues. They are activated by

Table 1. K+ channel families functionally associated with integrins. *List of the K+ channel families presently known to be physiologically related to integrin receptors. Table gives the standard names of genes and the corresponding subunits. The rightmost column lists some commonly used channel names. For details about ERG1a and ERG1b see reference 31.*

Channel Type—Subunit	Gene	Other Names
Voltage-Gated K+ Channels		
K_V 1.1-K_V 1.3	KCNA1-KCNA3	Delayed rectifiers
K_V 1.4	KCNA4	A-type
K_V 1.5-K_V 1.7	KCNA5-KCNA7	Delayed rectifiers
K_V 1.8	KCNA10	"
K_V 4.1-K_V 4.3	KCND1-KCND3	A-type
K_V 10.1	KCNH1	EAG 1
K_V 10.2	KCNH5	EAG 2
K_V 11.1a (splice variant)	KCNH2	ERG 1a
1b (splice variant)		ERG 1b
K_V 11.2	KCNH6	ERG 2
K_V 11.3	KCNH7	ERG 3
Inwardly Rectifying K+ Channels		IRK, GIRK, IR
Kir 1.1	KCNJ1	
Kir 2.1	KCNJ2	
Kir 2.2	KCNJ12	
Kir 2.3	KCNJ4	
Kir 2.4	KCNJ14	
Kir 3.1	KCNJ3	
Kir 3.2	KCNJ6	
Kir 3.3	KCNJ9	
Kir 3.4	KCNJ5	
Kir 4.1	KCNJ10	
Kir 4.2	KCNJ15	
Kir 5.1	KCNJ16	
Kir 6.1	KCNJ8	
Kir 6.2	KCNJ11	
Kir 7.1	KCNJ13	
Calcium Activated K+ Channels		
K_{Ca} 1.1	KCNMA1	BK, Slo
K_{Ca} 2.1-K_{Ca} 2.3	KCNN1-KCNN3	$SK_{Ca}1$-$SK_{Ca}3$
K_{Ca} 3.1	KCNN4	$IK_{Ca}1$
K_{Ca} 4.1	KCNT1	Slack, Slo2.2
K_{Ca} 4.2	KCNT2	Slick, Slo2.1
K_{Ca} 5.1	KCNU1	Slo3

$[Ca^{2+}]_i$, with EC_{50} around 500 nM. Activation is not caused by Ca^{2+} binding directly to the channel, but is mediated by calmodulin, which is tightly bound to each subunit. SK have γ around 10 pS and present inward rectification because of block produced by intracellular divalent cations.

K_{Ca} subunits are expressed in different tissues. BK usually controls the action potential afterhyperpolarization driven by Ca^{2+} influx and thus firing frequency. The role of other large-conductance

Introduction to Ion Channels 17

Table 2. Voltage-dependent Ca²⁺ channels. List of the voltage-gated Ca²⁺ channel types known to date. Table gives the subunit and gene symbols, plus some common names.

Subunit	Gene	Common Names
Main Subunit		
Ca$_V$ 1.1 (α_{1S})	CACNA1S	L, HVA
Ca$_V$ 1.2 (α_{1C})	CACNA1C	L, HVA
Ca$_V$ 1.3 (α_{1D})	CACNA1D	L, HVA
Ca$_V$ 1.4 (α_{1F})	CACNA1F	L, HVA
Ca$_V$ 2.1 (α_{1A})	CACNA1A	N, HVA
Ca$_V$ 2.2 (α_{1B})	CACNA1B	P/Q, HVA
Ca$_V$ 2.3 (α_{1E})	CACNA1E	R, HVA
Ca$_V$ 3.1 (α_{1G})	CACNA1G	T, LVA
Ca$_V$ 3.2 (α_{1H})	CACNA1H	T, LVA
Ca$_V$ 3.3 (α_{1I})	CACNA1I	T, LVA
Accessory Subunits		
$\alpha_2\delta_1$-$\alpha_2\delta_4$	CACNA2D1-CACNA2D4	
β_1-β_4	CACNB1-CACNB4	
γ_1-γ_8	CACNG1-CACNG8	

channels is less clear. IK and SK are widely distributed and their function are rather diversified, ranging from control of neuronal firing, to vascular tone regulation and control of cell proliferation.

Voltage-Gated Ca²⁺ Channels

Ca²⁺ influx through the plasma membrane controls cardiac and smooth muscle contraction, exocytosis, cell proliferation, motility and many other processes. Voltage-gated Ca²⁺ channels are activated by membrane depolarization. Broadly speaking, three functional categories can be distinguished (Table 2).[39,40] High-threshold Ca²⁺ channels activate around −30 mV and produce steady currents, with slow inactivation (L currents, from 'long lasting'). They typically trigger contraction in muscle and secretion in endocrine cells. In particular, they are responsible for the long depolarized plateau of the cardiac action potential. They can also regulate intracellular processes that converge on gene expression control. The second subfamily comprises N, P/Q and R currents. These also activate at relatively depolarized V_m and typically trigger neurotransmitter release, when activated by action potential invading the presynaptic terminal. Low-threshold Ca²⁺ currents (T currents, from 'transient') activate around −60 mV and present a much quicker inactivation. They usually control intrinsic cell firing, for example in the senoatrial node (the cardiac pacemaker) and thalamocortical neurons (which generate oscillatory bursting during slow-wave sleep). T currents are also named LVA (low voltage activated), whereas the other Ca²⁺ currents are sometimes collectively labeled as HVA (high voltage activated).

Cl⁻ Channels

Voltage-gated Cl⁻ channels are formed by two identical CLC-type subunits. To date, seven subunits are known (CLC-1 to CLC-7, corresponding to the genes *CLCN1* to *CLCN7*)[41], each containing an independent pore permeable to anions. The first high-resolution structure for a Cl⁻ channels was obtained in 2002.[9] CLC-3, CLC-4 and CLC-5 are expressed on intracellular vescicles, where they contribute to the control of pH and volume. The same may apply to CLC-6 and CLC-7, which cannot be expressed in heterologous systems. The other CLC's belong to the subfamily of muscle-type CLC channels. They are activated by depolarization and regulate the resting potential (especially in excitable cells), transepithelial flow and osmotic equilibrium in response to cell swelling.[41]

Cl⁻ channels activated by Ca^{2+} are also known to be expressed in a variety of cell types.[42] In mammals, their physiological roles range from sensory transduction to epithelial secretion and control of neuronal excitability. In some species, Ca^{2+}-activated Cl⁻ channels contribute to the repolarization of cardiac action potential. Their role in smooth muscle has been widely studied. When $[Ca^{2+}]_i$ increases, Cl⁻ channel activation depolarizes the cell, thus stimulating voltage-gated Ca^{2+} channels. In this way, Cl⁻ channels participate to the control of muscle contraction. Their role in vascular endothelial cells is still unclear. Unfortunately, the molecular identity of Ca^{2+}-activated Cl⁻ channels is still poorly known. From the present book's perspective, the CLCA protein family is interesting because these proteins have high omology to cell adhesion proteins and have been implicated in metastatic processes.[43] It is however still unclear whether CLCA are indeed Cl⁻ channels, or are subunits contributing to the Ca^{2+}-activated Cl⁻ channel structure, or perhaps modulatory proteins.[42]

Neurotransmitter-Gated Channels

Neurotransmitters can produce their effects by binding to pre, post or extrasynaptic receptors. These can be ion channels (ionotropic receptors) or receptors that activate intracellular signaling pathways (metabotropic receptors). Recent work (reviewed in Chapter 9) points to functional relations between integrin receptors and ionotropic receptors, particularly nAChRs and glutamate receptors, whose main features we briefly describe (Table 3).

The muscular nAChR is an heteropentamer $(\alpha 1)_2 \beta 1 \delta \varepsilon$ (γ in the embryo) that mediates neuromuscular transmission. It fully activates when two ACh molecules bind to the specific extracellular pockets mostly (but not exclusively) formed by residues belonging to the α subunits. As to the neuronal nAChRs, twelve subunits are known: $\alpha 2$-$\alpha 10$ and $\beta 2$-$\beta 4$.[44] The role of the different subunits is only partially understood. A9 and $\alpha 10$ are mainly expressed in the cochlea. In the central nervous system, both homo- and heteropentameric receptors are thought to be expressed. The former are probably mostly $(\alpha 7)_5$, whereas the spectrum of heteropentamers is much wider.

Table 3. Ligand-gated channels functionally associated with integrins. Table gives the names of subunits and genes, for the indicated nicotinic and glutamate receptors.

Channel Type	Gene	Subunit
Nicotinic Receptors		
muscular AChR	CHRNA1	$\alpha 1$
	CHRNB1	$\beta 1$
	CHRND	δ
	CHRNE	ε
	CHRNG	γ
neuronal AChR	CHRNA2-CHRNA1	$\alpha 2$-$\alpha 10$
	CHRNB2-CHRNB4	$\beta 2$-$\beta 4$
Glutamate Receptors		
NMDA Receptor	GRIN1	NR1
	GRIN2A-GRIN2D	NR2A-NR2D
	GRIN3A-GRIN3B	NR3A-NR3B
AMPA Receptor	GRIA1-GRIA4	GluR1-GluR4
Kainate Receptor	GRIK1-GRIK3	GluR5-GluR7
	GRIK4-GRIK5	KA-1-KA-2

Among these, a common form is $(\alpha 4)_2(\beta 2)_3$, at least in rodents, whereas in the peripheral nervous system α3 and β4 subunits are widespread.[44] Nicotinic receptors are permeable to Na^+, K^+ and Ca^{2+}. The permeability to the latter is variable, but particularly pronounced in α7-containing receptors. In peripheral ganglia, nAChRs mediate postsynaptic transmission. In the brain, presynaptic nAChRs regulate transmitter release, but postsynaptic roles have also been observed. In general, cholinergic transmission in the brain controls the level of arousal with implications for learning and for the transitions between sleep and waking phases.[45]

Glutamate is the main excitatory transmitter, in the CNS. Three families of ionotropic glutamate receptors are known, pharmacologically distinguishable by three relatively specific agonists: N-methyl-D-aspartate (NMDA), α-amino-3-hydroxy-5-methyl-4-isoxazole propionic acid (AMPA) and kainate (KA).[46,47] Channels gated by AMPA and KA are also named nonNMDA receptors. In the presence of glutamate, they activate very quickly and then desensitize within about 30 ms. NonNMDA receptors are expressed in most central neurons, in which they generate the early large component of excitatory postsynaptic currents. They are usually permeable to Na^+ and K^+, but not Ca^{2+}. The NMDA receptors open and close relatively slowly, compared to the nonNMDA and thus carry the slow component of the excitatory postsynaptic currents. They require extracellular glycine for opening, in the presence of glutamate. In addition, at negative V_m they are inhibited by extracellular Mg^{2+}. Hence, when glutamate is released onto a resting neuron, NMDA channels do not carry significant current until the membrane is sufficiently depolarized (e.g., by nonNMDA receptors). NMDA receptors are permeable to Ca^{2+} as well as to Na^+ and K^+. Overall, these features produce at least two physiological consequences. First, when a neuron is sufficiently depolarized by intense presynaptic release, NMDA receptor activation leads to significant Ca^{2+} influx. This stimulates intracellular pathways with ensuing effects on long-lasting synaptic remodeling. Activity-dependent synaptic modifications are intensely studied because of possible implications for learning and memory processes. Second, persistent levels of extracellular glutamate may have neurotoxic effects (excitotoxicity) because steady Ca^{2+} influx activate intracellular pathways that may lead to cell death. Ionotropic glutamate receptors are also expressed in many non-excitable cells, such as astrocytes, lymphocytes, endocrine cells and some tumours. In general however, the nonneural glutamate functions are still matter of debate.[48]

Conclusion

By coupling the patch-clamp technique with the modern molecular biological methods allows to study ion channels in living cells with great sophistication. Most of the channel families known to date have been found to be implicated in integrin-dependent signaling. The subsequent chapters illustrate some of the best studied examples in this new and promising research field.

Acknowledgements

The present work was supported by the University of Milano-Bicocca (FAR program), the Fondazione Banca del Monte Lombardia and a fellowship to CDR from the Ingenio Program of Regione Lombardia.

References

1. Hodgkin AL, Huxley AF. A quantitative description of membrane current and its application to conduction and excitation in nerve. J Physiol 1952; 117:500-544.
2. Skou JC. The influence of some cations on an adenosine triphosphatase from peripheral nerves. Biochem Biophys Acta 1957; 23:394-401.
3. Eccles JC. The physiology of synapses. New York: Academic Press, 1964.
4. Katz B. The release of neural transmitter substances. Liverpool University Press, 1969.
5. Conti F, Wanke E. Channel noise in nerve membranes and lipid bilayers. Q Rev Biophys 1975; 8:451-506.
6. Robinson JD. Mechanisms of Synaptic Transmission. Bridging the Gaps (1890-1990). Oxford University Press, 2001.
7. Noda M, Takahashi H, Tanabe T et al. Primary structure of the α-subunit precursor of Torpedo californica acetylcholine receptor deduced from cDNA sequence. Nature 1982; 299:793-797.

8. Doyle DA, Morais-Cabral J, Pfuetzner RA et al. The structure of the potassium channel: molecular basis of K^+ conduction and selectivity. Science 1998; 280:69-77.
9. Dutzler R, Campbell EB, Cadene M et al. X-ray structure of a CLC chloride channel at 3.0 Å reveals the molecular basis of anion selectivity. Nature 2002; 415:287-294.
10. Neher E, Sakmann B. Single-channel currents recorded from membrane of denervated frog muscle fibres. Nature 1976; 260:799-802.
11. Hamill OP, Marty E, Neher B et al. Improved patch-clamp techniques for high-resolution current recording from cells and cell-free membrane patches. Pflügers Arch 1981; 391:85-100.
12. Aidley DJ, The Physiology of Excitable Cells, 3rd Ed. Cambridge University Press, 1998.
13. Blaustein MP, Kao JPY, Matteson DR. Cellular Physiology. Elsevier Inc, 2004;
14. Johnston D, Wu SM. Foundations of cellular neurophysiology. MIT Press 1995.
15. Hille B. Ion channels of excitable membranes. Sinauer Associates 2001.
16. Somjen GC. Ions in the Brain: Normal Function, Seizures and Stroke. Oxford University Press, 2004.
17. Ben-Ari Y, Gaiarsa JL, Tyzio R et al. GABA: a pioneer transmitter that excites immature neurons and generates primitive oscillations. Physiol Rev 2007; 87:1215-1284.
18. Gutman GA, Chandy KG, Grissmer S et al. International Union of Pharmacology. LIII. Nomenclature and molecular relationships of voltage-gated potassium channels. Pharmacol Rev 2005; 57:473-508.
19. McKinnon R, Yellen G. Mutations affecting TEA blockade and ion permeation in voltage-activated K^+ channels. Science 1990; 250:276-279.
20. Yool AJ, Schwartz TL. Alteration of ionic selectivity of a K^+ channel. Nature 1991; 349:700-704.
21. Bucossi G, Eismann E, Sesti F et al. Time-dependent current decline in cyclic GMP-gated bovine channels caused by point mutations in the pore region expressed in Xenopus oocytes. J Physiol 1996; 493:409-441.
22. Becchetti A, Gamel K, Torre V. Cyclic nucleotide-gated channels. Pore topology studied through the accessibility of reporter cysteines. J Gen Physiol 1999; 114:377-392.
23. Liu J, Siegelbaum SA. Change of pore helix conformational state upon opening of cyclic nucleotide-gated channels. Neuron 2000; 28:899-909.
24. Chittajallu R, Chen Y, Wang H et al. Regulation of Kv1 subunit expression in oligodendrocyte progenitor cells and their role in G_1/S phase progression of the cell cycle. Proc Natl Acad Sci USA 2002; 99:2350-2355.
25. Zhou M, Kimelberg HK. Freshly isolated astrocytes from rat hippocampus show two distinct current patterns and different $[K^+]_o$ uptake capabilities. J Neurophysiol 2000; 84:2746-2757.
26. Smith PL, Baukrowitz T, Yellen G. The inward rectification mechanism of the HERG cardiac potassium channel. Nature 1996; 379:833-836.
27. Sanguinetti MC, Tristani-Firouzi P. hERG potassium channels and cardiac arrhythmia. Nature 2006; 440:463-469.
28. Guasti L, Cilia E, Crociani O et al. Expression pattern of the Ether-à-go-go-related (ERG) family proteins in the adult mouse central nervous system: evidence for coassembly of different subunits. J Comp Neurol 2005; 491:157-174.
29. Arcangeli A, Becchetti A. Ion channels and the cell cycle. In: D. Janigro, ed. The Cell Cycle in the Nervous Central System. Hartford:Humana Press, 2006.
30. Morais Cabral JH, Lee A, Cohen SL et al. Crystal structure and functional analysis of the HERG potassium channel N terminus: a eukaryotic PAS domain. Cell 1998; 95:649-655.
31. London B, Trudeau MC, Newton KP et al. Two isoforms of the mouse ether-à-go-go-related gene coassemble to form channels with properties similar to the rapidly activating component of the cardiac delayed rectifier K^+ current. Circ Res 1997; 81:870-878.
32. Crociani O, Guasti L, Balzi M et al. Cell cycle-dependent expression of HERG1 and HERG1b isoforms in tumor cells. J Biol Chem 2003; 278:2947-2955.
33. Lu Z. Mechanisms of rectification in inward-rectifier K^+ channels. Annu Rev Physiol 2004; 66:103-129.
34. Nichols CG, Lopatin AN. Inward rectifier potassium channels. Annu Rev Physiol 1997; 59:171-191.
35. Kubo Y, Adelman JP, Clapham DE et al. International Union of Pharmacology. LIV nomenclature and molecular relationships of inwardly rectifying potassium channels. Pharmacol Rev 2005; 57:509-526.
36. Stocker M. Ca^{2+}-activated K^+ channels: molecular determinants and function of the SK family. Nat Rev Neurosci 2004; 5:758-770.
37. Salkoff L, Butler A, Ferreira G et al. High-conductance potassium channels of the SLO family. Nat Rev Neurosci 2006; 5:921-931.
38. Wei AD, Gutman GA, Aldrich R et al. International Union of Pharmacology. LII nomenclature and molecular relationships of calcium-activated potassium channels. Pharmacol Rev 2005; 57:463-472.
39. Khosravani H, Zamponi GW. Voltage-gated calcium channels and idiopathic generalized epilepsies. Physiol Rev 2006; 86:941-966.

40. Catterall WA, Perez-Royes E, Snutch TP et al. International Union of Pharmacology. XLVIII nomenclature and structure-function relationships of voltage-gated calcium channels. Pharmacol Rev 2005; 57:411-425.
41. Chen T-Y. Structure and function of CLC channels. Annu Rev Physiol 2005; 67:809-839.
42. Hartzell C, Putzier I, Arreola J. Calcium-activated chloride channels. Annu Rev Physiol 2005; 67:719-758.
43. Abdel-Ghany M, Cheng H-C, Eible RC et al. Focal adhesion kinase activated by β_4 integrin ligation to mCLCA1 mediates early metastatic growth. J Biol Chem 2002; 277:34391-34400.
44. Gotti C, Clementi F. Neuronal nicotinic receptors: from structure to pathology. Prog Neurobiol 2004; 74:363-396.
45. Dani JA, Bertrand D. Nicotinic acetylcholine receptors and nicotinic cholinergic mechanisms of the central nervous system. Annu Rev Pharmacol Toxicol 2007; 47:699-729.
46. Mayer ML, Armstrong N. Structure and function of glutamate receptor ion channels. Annu Rev Physiol 2004; 66:161-181.
47. Mayer ML. Glutamate receptor ion channels. Curr Opin Neurobiol 2005; 15:282-288.
48. Nedergaard M, Takano T, Hansen AJ. Beyond the role of glutamate as a neurotransmitter. Nat Rev Neurosci 2002; 3:748-753.

CHAPTER 3

Biochemical Methods to Study the Interactions Between Integrins and Ion Channels

Olivia Crociani*

Abstract

Protein-protein interactions between integrins and ion channels consist in a complicated bidirectional talk, not yet understood in detail, which triggers a downstream signaling network. Such a coordinated process occurs in discrete, localized microcompartments and involves different membrane and cytoplasmic proteins. Since the early nineties, when the first functional association between integrins and ion channels was characterized, the number of similar examples is constantly increasing. Identifying the components of this pathway has general importance for cell physiology and will eventually lead to fully understand the role of ion channels in the physiological processes typically controlled by integrin receptors, such as cell adhesion, migration and proliferation.

Here, we detail the main experimental methods currently available to study these processes and discuss their advantages and disadvantages. Biochemical copurification and genetic interaction studies, as well as high-throughput screening, can be performed to initially identify the interacting proteins. Successively, in vitro binding assays such as pull-down and immunoprecipitation-based techniques allow to verify and better characterize these partnerships, possibly in combination with mass spectrometry methods.

When transient interactions are involved, more sophisticated techniques, such as photoaffinity labeling procedures, are necessary to detect the multiprotein complexes by having them covalently bound together as they interact. To provide even more thorough analyses of the formation, function and composition of protein complexes, other technologies such as confocal microscopy, fluorescence resonance energy transfer microscopy and site directed mutagenesis (possibly in murine models) have to be performed.

The progressive accumulation of data defining novel protein protein interactions has been considerably accelerated by the identification of specific sequence motifs that regulate integrin binding to other proteins as well as integrin recognition sequences in the ligand. Moreover, the availability of protein tagging strategies and the increased sensitivity of mass spectrometry-based methods for protein identification have also contributed important tools. In the near future, the coupling of traditional techniques with proteomic approaches is likely to offer invaluable help in unraveling integrin-ion channel interactions, thus elucidating the biological implication of these complexes.

*Olivia Crociani—Department of Experimental Pathology and Oncology, University of Firenze. Viale G.B. Morgagni 50, 50134 Firenze, Italy. Email: olivia.crociani@unifi.it

Integrins and Ion Channels: Molecular Complexes and Signaling, edited by Andrea Becchetti and Annarosa Arcangeli. ©2010 Landes Bioscience and Springer Science+Business Media.

Introduction

During the last fifteen years, there have been numerous reports of direct and indirect functional interactions between integrin receptors and ion channels.[1] The presence, in a given protein, of specific peptide sequences that typically mediate integrin interaction is usually a first hint that such an interaction occurs.[2] However, demonstrating that a specific protein-protein complex is indeed formed during some cellular process requires extensive evidence obtained with a series of independent experimental procedures. In fact, ambiguous results are easily obtained, especially when the interacting partner is expressed at low levels, as is often the case with ion channels. The problem is sometimes so severe that the genuine partners have to be identified among very many spurious ones. For example, Selbach and Mann showed that after co-immunoprecipitation (IP), more than 95% of the identified proteins might be false positive interactors.[3] This critical issue highlights the necessity of good ways to validate the identified interaction partners.

In this chapter, we stress the idea that a well-done characterization of protein-protein interactions is necessary for a thorough understanding of the relationship between integrins and ion channels. Traditionally, protein identities are obtained by yeast two hybrid screening or biochemical copurification and then commonly characterized by co-IP, pull down assay and immunoblotting. Moreover, protein colocalization is determined by confocal microscopic analyses or other fluorescence-based/enzyme-mediated reactions.[4,5] More recently, the identification of protein-protein interactions has taken advantage of both genetic and biochemical 'traps'. Different genetic tools are in fact available for identifying molecular interactions among proteins. These methods need to be supplemented by molecular and/or cellular approaches to confirm that the putative multiprotein complexes do occur in living cells. Moreover, functional assays are necessary to assess their physiological relevance in the cellular and tissual context.

It is not however mandatory that the identification of a specific interaction is carried out by screening methods. Alternative procedures may involve a well-done characterization by using traditional or novel techniques. In particular, many recent experimental approaches, such as the yeast three hybrid system, protein arrays and photoaffinity labeling, do now permit to collect the multiple line of evidence necessary to build up a convincing case for the biological significance of the functional and/or physical interaction between different types of membrane proteins.

Interaction studies involving ion channels are a great challenge for the future, because they are essential to understand the relation between the many physiological mechanisms mediated by channel proteins and the extracellular environment. The concourse of established methods as well as procedures still in course of refinement will definitely be necessary to obtain a full picture of this topic, which is particularly hard to elucidate because ion channels are not only scarcely soluble, as is typical of integral membrane proteins, but are also often expressed at low surface density.

Yeast Two-Hybrid Screening

This method is one of the most commonly used to study protein–protein interactions.[6] It uses the transcription process to make predictions about protein interaction. The yeast two-hybrid system is based on the ability of an interacting protein pair (Fig. 1A, Protein a and b) to bring together the DNA-binding domain (BD) and the activation domain (AD) of a transcription factor in vivo, so as to stimulate the transcription of a reporter gene that thus signals the occurrence of the interaction between the two proteins. In brief, a protein of interest is fused to a DNA-BD (BD-a) and transfected in a yeast host cell bearing a reporter gene, able to respond to the full transcription factor (BD+AD). Therefore, the fusion protein containing the DNA-BD cannot activate transcription in the absence of the proper AD. It is instead used as a "bait" or as a "target" to screen a library of cDNA clones, that are fused to the AD. The DNA clones that encode proteins capable of forming protein-protein interactions with the bait, are identified by virtue of their ability to cause activation of the reporter gene. Therefore, the yeast two-hybrid system is devised to identify those genes that encode proteins physically associated with a given protein, in vivo.[7] In the case of ion channels, the intracellular C terminus seems generally to be the best suited portion to perform a yeast two-hybrid experiment.[8]

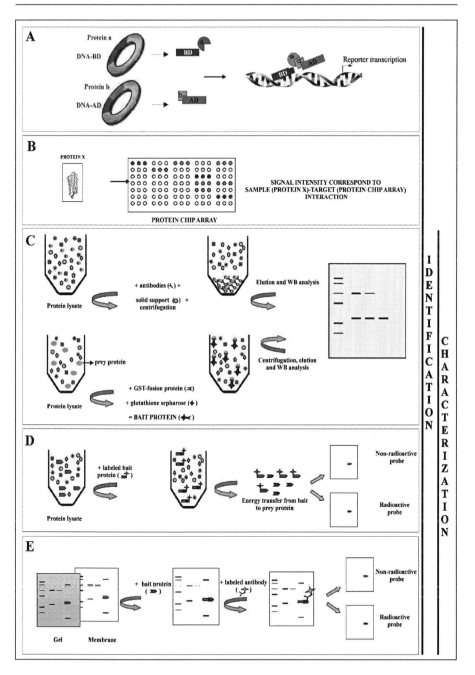

Figure 1. Different approaches used to identify and/or characterize new protein-protein complexes. A) yeast two hybrid system; B) protein array; C) affinity-based techniques: co-IP (upper panel) and pull-down assay (lower panel); D) photoaffinity labeling; E) Far Western Blot. For details see text.

Many established protein interactions were first suggested by application of this method, which is a quite simple procedure, provided that one has the cDNAs of interest (full length or partial). This technique can be used to perform wide library screening for potential partners of a certain protein, as it allows to detect even weak interactions. However, it also presents some disadvantages. First, it cannot work if the protein-protein interaction under study requires some posttranslational modification that does not occur in yeast. This drawback has been recently circumvented by the development of "yeast tri-hybrid" systems, whereby the appropriate modifying enzyme is co-expressed in the yeast cell.[9] Second, some mammalian proteins are toxic for yeast, which is especially unfortunate when screening libraries. Finally, false positive interactions may appear. To avoid these problems, parallel high-throughput approaches (Fig. 1B) are now possible by carrying out proteome-wide interaction screens (by using for example protein arrays, as will be discussed below). These can of course be also applied to the study of integrin-channel interaction or ion channel regulation.[10]

Affinity-Based Screening: IP Assays

To validate the results obtained by methods for identifying protein-protein interaction, it is always recommendable to perform supplementary assays in vitro. These are based on the natural affinity of binding partners for each other and are widely adopted for both interaction discovery and confirmation. The experimental strategies can be direct or indirect: in the latter case, binding is mediated by an antibody against a target antigen, that in turn precipitates an interacting protein.

Among these methods, a most widely used is based on the IP assay. A specific monoclonal or polyclonal antibody against a certain target antigen is allowed to form an immune complex in a sample, such as a total or a membrane-enriched lysate. The immune complex is then combined with an insoluble particle or bead coupled either with Protein A (a protein originally isolated from *Staphilococcus aureus*) or Protein G (protein expressed in group C and G of streptococcal bacteria), so as to be immobilized and precipitated. Any protein not immobilized and precipitated by the support coated with Protein A or G is subsequently washed away. Finally, the immune complex (both antigen and antibody) are eluted from the support by boiling the sample in a reducing buffer and analyzed by SDS-PolyAcrylamide Gel Electrophoresis (PAGE), often followed by Western blot (WB) tests, to verify the identity of the antigen.

Traditionally, the immune complex formation is preceded by a preclearing step, in which the protein lysate is incubated with Protein A or G in absence of antibodies. This step is needed to lower the amount of non specific contaminants in the sample and is recommended when the protein of interest is poorly expressed on the membrane surface.

The choice of a specific protocol to perform an efficient IP is always critical. When studying the interaction between integrins and ion channels, it is advisable to prolong the antigen-antibody binding step up to 16 hours and to reduce the incubation time with Protein A or G to no more than 2 hours. In this way, the immune complex formation is stimulated, whereas the aspecific binding to the solid support is minimized. Of course, the success of any IP protocol strictly depends on the affinity of the antibody for its antigen, as well as for the solid support. Polyclonal antibodies are usually more suitable for this assay, compared to the monoclonals, because of the multiple epitopes recognized, which increases the avidity of the antibody. Furthermore, a monoclonal antibody presents a more variable strength of interaction to Protein A or G with respect to a polyclonal one, depending on isotype. Such a factor is fundamental when choosing the more appropriate protein to isolate the antigen-antibody complex. It is worth noting that Protein G binds well to most subclasses of rat and mouse Immunoglobulin (Ig), whereas Protein A is more affine to the mouse subclasses IgG2a, IgG2b and IgG3. Finally, it is important not to use the same antibody to immunoprecipitate and decorate the subsequent WB, to avoid very high background signals.[11] The usual method to validate, characterize, or confirm a specific protein-protein interaction involves co-IP (Fig. 1C, upper panel). In this case, the target antigen that is precipitated by the antibody coprecipitates a binding partner (or protein complex), from the lysate. In detail, the interacting protein is bound to the target antigen, which is then bound by the antibody, that finally binds the Protein A or Protein G on their gel support. The usual assumption behind these studies is that the proteins that coprecipitate with the target antigen are also functionally related to it, although it should be kept in mind that proving this assumption requires supplementary physiological tests. A most commonly encountered problem with IP tests is the very high background signal. This problem arises when the same antibody (or an antibody from the same species) is used in both IP and WB, since the heavy (H, 55 kDa) and light chains (L, 25 kDa) of the antibody employed are also eluted from the beads and then subsequently size-fractionated by SDS-PAGE with the antigen.[11] In this case, the secondary antibody used to detect the primary antibody on WBs will also recognize the H and L chain bands on WB filters. If the antigen size is comparable to that of these chains, its signal may be masked since the H and L chains are much more abundant. To circumvent this problem, a variety of strategies can be performed. One possibility is incubating the cells with ^{35}S-methionine and ^{35}S-cysteine, to be able to isotopically visualize the protein after IP and SDS-PAGE. This method is effective when the antigen is abundant and the antibody is specific and highly sensitive.[12] Alternatively, the primary antibody can be covalently crosslinked to Protein A- or Protein G-sepharose beads before IP.[13] Still other approaches exclude reducing agents from the IP buffers and avoid boiling the samples, in order to preserve the antibody tetrameric structure, which then migrates as a 160 kDa complex. The main limitation of this procedure is that in the absence of reducing agents and without heating, the antigen may not be effectively released from the antibody.

As mentioned above, the best strategy to avoid cross-reactivity is still performing WB with antibodies from different species, if such antibodies are available. Another possibility is the use of specific epitopes like HA- and c-Myc, as tags to be ligated to the protein under study. To this purpose, the protein is isolated as cDNA, the stop codon is removed and is ligated in a specific vector containing HA or c-Myc coding sequence, so that these tags are fused in frame to the 3' end of the protein itself. The commercially available high-affinity monoclonal antibodies anti-HA and anti-c-Myc, because of their excellent specificity allow to obtain a WB detection without sham signals.

All the procedures listed above have been indeed applied to the study of the interaction between integrins and ion channels. An example is given by the G protein-activated inward rectifier K⁺ (GIRK) channels. These proteins are the only known K⁺ channels that have an arginine-glycine-aspartate motif (the RGD site), a typical integrin-specific recognition site.[2] Co-IP of GIRK1 and GIRK4 with an endogenous β1A integrin subunit was in fact demonstrated in oocytes and mouse fibroblasts.[14,15] Further direct evidence for a physical association between channels and integrins exists for T-lymphocytes.[16] In these cells, co-IP tests with antibodies specific for each protein showed that Kv 1.3 channels and β1 integrins are bound. Other evidences of a physical link between ion channels and integrins have been recently reported. For example, the transient receptor potential vanilloid 4 (TRPV4) from cultured dorsal root ganglia neurons was immunoprecipitated with α2 integrin, which highlighted a specific 150 kDa band in WBs.[17] Similarly, a physical interaction between hERG1 K⁺ channels and β1 integrins has been initially demonstrated in neuroblastoma cells (SH SY5Y), by immunoprecipitating β1 and then revealing hERG1 with a specific antibody on WBs.[18,19] These results were also confirmed in a HEK 293 cell line over expressing hERG1, where the strict relation between the two proteins has been demonstrated by carrying out IP with an anti-β1, plus an anti-hERG1 for WB detection and vice versa.[19]

Pull-Down Assay

This is a further in vitro method used to determine the physical interaction between two or more proteins. Such technique is useful for both confirming the existence of a complex and as initial screening assay, for identifying unknown protein-protein interactions.

This approach is a form of affinity purification and is very similar to IP, except that a bait protein immobilized on a solid support (e.g., sepharose beads) is used instead of an antibody (Fig. 1C, lower panel). If the bait associates with a specific protein, after incubation in a cellular lysate, pelleting of the sample by centrifugation results in precipitation of the protein complex. Bound complexes can then be eluted, after proper washing to remove aspecific interactions.

Bait proteins for pull-down assays can be generated either by linking an affinity reactive tag to proteins purified by traditional methods (biotynilated bait proteins) or by expressing recombinant fusion-tagged proteins. Typically, in the latter case, the relevant parts of the bait protein are produced in bacteria as recombinant protein fused to Glutathione S-Transferase (GST) or 6X hystidine, after cloning the corresponding cDNA sequence in a specific vector. This procedure has been performed successfully to confirm the interaction between β4 integrin and the human proteins CLCA2 (hCLCA2).[20] Moreover, the pull down assay turned out to be a crucial method to clarify that the physical link between hERG1 and Rac1 proteins (demonstrated by a co-IP strategy) results in modulation of the small GTPase activity by the K^+ channel, thus suggesting that an ion channel mediates a key step in the integrin-regulated signaling.[19]

An advantage of the pull down assay is that it is efficient and easy to use. However, it has shortcomings as well. First, not all proteins can be easily over-expressed in a soluble form in bacteria; second, fusion proteins expressed in prokaryotic cells may lack the posttranslational modifications required for protein-protein interactions; finally, nonspecific binding can increase the occurrence of false positives.[21] To avoid such an undesirable background, carefully designed control experiments are absolutely necessary, for generating biologically significant results. A negative control, consisting of a nontreated affinity support (minus bait protein sample), helps to identify and eliminate the false positives caused by nonspecific binding of proteins to the affinity support. On the other hand, the immobilized bait control (plus bait protein sample, minus prey protein sample) helps to identify and eliminate the false positives caused by nonspecific binding of proteins to the tag of the bait protein.

Photoaffinity Labeling Techniques for Studying Transient Protein-Protein Interaction

The methods listed above target stable protein-protein interactions, but most of biological processes are based on transient protein-protein complexes. These are characterized by small contact areas and less defined conformational changes upon binding of the interacting protein.[22] Transient interactions are more conveniently confirmed by cross-linking or label transfer methods that allow to detect protein-protein complexes by linking the component proteins by covalent bonds, as they interact. When exposed to common cross-linkers, most of the functional groups react quickly enough to permit a 'freezing' in place of even transient or weak interactions, thus fixing the interacting molecules in a complex sufficiently stable for isolation and characterization. Traditional amine-reactive cross linkers such as formaldehyde or N-hydroxysuccinimide (NHS)-ester derivatives have been used to this purpose in vitro. Formaldehyde has been used extensively to reversibly cross-link proteins through primary amines with a juxtaposed bond distance. However, it spontaneously forms polymers in solution and is not protein-specific as it also cross-links proteins to DNA and other macromolecules. Bifunctional NHS-ester cross-linkers (e.g., disuccinimidyl glutarate and disuccinimidyl suberate) are more specific for proteins, but only cross-link specific amino acid residues at defined spacer lengths. Additionally, these compounds must be modified to permeate cell membranes for functioning and must be quenched to prevent excessive cross-linking.[23] To avoid these disadvantages, the use of photoreactive agents is preferred over methods that use standard bifunctional thermoreactive cross-linkers such as the above. These agents contain photoreactive groups that can be stimulated to react at selected times by UV light irradiation. Moreover, photoreactive cross-linkers limit the formation of conjugate polymer artefacts. However, a typical downside of the photoreactive coupling methods is that the yield of conjugate formation is usually low. Many aryl azide groups undergo a particularly inefficient ring-expansion reaction. This targets their reactivity exclusively toward amine groups and thus limits their utility for nonselective insertion into neighboring protein structures. In addition, the solvent reactions that quench the photoreactive moiety often exceed the reactions with a desired target. Some photoreactive groups, such as halogen-substituted aryl azides and benzophenones, have much better conjugation yields and can efficiently capture interacting molecules. Cross linkers that incorporate a perfluoroazidobenzamido group, for instance, do not undergo ring expansion after photolyzing. Thus, on UV exposure, they produce a highly reactive nitrene that effectively couples to any protein structures nearby. For more details, see the "Pierce protein interaction handbook," available online (www.piercenet.com).

A related method is named 'label transfer' and involves cross-linking interacting molecules (e.g., bait and prey proteins) with a labeled cross-linking agent. The linkage between bait and prey is then cleaved, so that the label remains attached to the prey (Fig. 1D). In this way, a label can be transferred from a given protein to an unknown interactor. The label can then be used to purify and/or detect the interacting protein. Label transfer is particularly valuable because of its ability to identify proteins that interact weakly or transiently with the protein of interest. New non-isotopic reagents (labeled with biotin, instead of ^{125}I) and new methods continue to make this technique more accessible and simple to perform.[24]

Photoaffinity labeling techniques, in particular cross-linking protocols, have been crucial to establish membrane localization and assembly of ion channels. They have clarified some controversial results obtained by other procedures and, overall, represent very important tools to study the ion channel organization and interaction with other proteins.[25]

Far Western Blot Analysis (Far WB)

This method aims at studying the effect of posttranslational modifications on protein-protein interactions, examining the interaction sequences using synthetic peptides as probes and identifying protein-protein interactions, without using antigen-specific antibodies. It involves immobilization of the prey proteins of interest on a two dimensional surface, followed by incubation with the bait protein (Fig. 1E). The subsequent detection of the bait protein is typically carried out with a labeled antibody.[26] For its characteristics, Far-WB procedures must be performed with care to preserve as much as possible the native conformation and interaction conditions of the proteins under study. Denatured proteins may not be able to interact, resulting in a failure to identify an interaction. Alternatively, proteins presented in nonnative conformations may interact in artifactual ways, which results in spurious interactions.

This procedure has been used to confirm a partnership involving β4 integrin and hCLCA2 protein.[27] To this purpose, after subjecting the SDS-PAGE resolved and the blotted β4 integrin to denaturing and renaturing cycles, blots were probed with Myc-tagged hCLCA2. The hCLCA2-binding to β4 was then visualized by anti-Myc antibodies. Results, showing an interaction between the two proteins, were also validated by probing blot-immobilized Myc-tagged hCLCA2 with soluble β4 integrin and then incubating the membrane with an anti-β4 integrin.

High-Throughput Protein-Protein Interaction Analysis, Followed by Validation of Candidate Interactors through Different Experimental Approaches

Protein chip arrays involve immobilization of bait proteins onto a chip surface, followed by exposure to potential prey proteins (Fig. 1B, PROTEIN X) and detection of interactions through mass spectrometry, colorimetric detection or other characterization methods.[28] Briefly, protein microarrays consist of antibodies, proteins, protein fragments, peptides, aptamers or carbohydrate elements, that are coated or immobilized in a grid-like pattern. The arrayed molecules are then used to screen and assess the patterns of interaction with samples containing distinct proteins or classes of proteins.

Similar protocols have been applied to identify specific integrin-ion channel interactions, exploiting motifs known to critically regulate the protein-protein partnership involving integrins. A typical experiment based on this approach is described in ref. 10, which provides the first demonstration of an association between the nucleotide-sensitive chloride channel ICln and the αIIbβ3 integrin, identified by screening a high density protein array with a biotin-tagged conserved integrin aminoacid sequence.

The availability of such biological sequences, as well as the presence of integrin recognition sequences in the ligand, has accelerated the accumulation of data defining novel protein-protein interactions. These studies have also benefited from the availability of protein tagging methods and the increased sensitivity of mass spectrometry applied to protein identification.

The main integrin-binding motif is RGD, but many other bioactive peptides bind to the majority of integrins.[2] Such motifs can be used as essential tools to validate an "interactome" and many examples have been reported since the early 1990's, when, for the first time, synthetic peptides competing with specific integrin ligands were used to alter the integrin-ion channel interactions.[29] In this regard, the physiological consequences of the integrin-channel interaction have been determined by studying the intracellular responses produced by extracellular application of these peptides and their inhibition after site-specific mutation of the corresponding ligand domain.[29] Conversely, application of the peptide followed by the lack of competition with the integrin-ligand motif presented by a specific channel (i.e., persistent co-IP capacity) has been a crucial step to rule out the presence of a physical interaction between the two molecules.[15] Examples of direct interaction between integrins and ion channels have also been disclosed by the use of commercially available monoclonal antibodies and/or specific inhibitors capable of blocking or activating both molecules.[30,31]

Conclusion: Past and Future Application of Biochemical Approaches to Characterize the Interactions between Integrins and Ion Channels

As pointed out in the previous chapters and resumed in Figure 1, the mechanisms of interaction between integrins and ion channels have to be studied by applying different biochemical approaches. Upon adhesion to specific ligands (typically extracellular proteins) integrins become active and can associate with ion channels. This physical interaction can be identified by yeast two-hybrid screening or other kinds of affinity-based screening (e.g., pull-down assay) and then confirmed in vivo by co-IP and double-label immunofluorescence. The latter procedure is a frequently employed method to evidence that proteins are in the same subcellular location (a prerequisite to demonstrate a direct interaction), but these results can be further confirmed by more sophisticated optical methods, as discussed in the following chapter.

Furthermore, integrin engagement leads to the activation of downstream signaling proteins (such as FAK and Src kinases and G proteins), which, besides stimulating cellular responses, can activate ion channels by phosphorylation or other mechanisms. In the same way, ion channels themselves can activate integrins or downstream signaling by modulating ion flow or perhaps direct conformational coupling. Therefore, all of the biochemical procedures outlined in the present review can be applied to identify the different members of the intricated and still poorly understood, downstream network stimulated by integrin-channel interaction.[1] It is worth noting that the traditional methods of protein analysis are inadequate to fully characterize and understand these structures, which contain many components and are highly dynamic.[32] In fact, many components of the signal transduction networks interact with each other through weak or transient interactions.[33] As mentioned earlier, in vivo chemical cross-linking is an attractive approach to "cement" weak and transient protein-protein interactions. However, to avoid false positive and false negative results, new proteomics technologies should be applied to distinguish specific from nonspecific interactions, rapidly and sensitively. Such procedures are being developed in different laboratories and are based on a specific tagging at the aminoacid or peptide level, with radioisotopes or fluorescence dyes, subsequently resolved by mass spectrometry or two dimensional electrophoresis.[34] In addition, highly sensitive phosphoprotein dyes to detect phosphoserine-, posphothreonine- and phosphotyrosine-containing proteins directly onto SDS-PAGE gels and two-dimensional gels have recently become commercially available. These are fully compatible with subsequent mass spectrometry analysis. No doubt, all of these procedures, already considered fundamental tools in the signal transduction field, will play a major role in the integration of biochemical information with higher-order biological systems and will determine important progresses in elucidating the signaling cascades involving ion channels in a tissue context.

Acknowledgements

This work has been supported by grants from the Associazione Italiana per la Ricerca sul Cancro (AIRC), the Association for International Cancer Research (AICR), the Ministero dell'Università e della Ricerca Scientifica e Tecnologica (PRIN 2005), the Associazione Genitori Noi per Voi and the Ente Cassa di Risparmio di Firenze.

References

1. Arcangeli A, Becchetti A. Complex functional interaction between integrin receptors and ion channels. Trends Cell Biol 2006; 16:631-9.
2. Rouslahti E. RGD and other recognition sequences for integrins. Annu Rev Cell Dev Biol 1996; 12:697-715.
3. Selbach M., Mann M. Protein interaction screening by quantitative immunoprecipitation combined with knockdown (QUICK). Nat Methods 2006; 3:981-83.
4. Morell M, Espargaró A, Avilés FX et al. Detection of transient protein-protein interactions by bimolecular fluorescence complementation: The Antibodyl-SH3 case. Proteomics 2007; 7:1023-36.
5. Kotani N, Gu J, Isaji T et al. Biochemical visualization of cell surface molecular clustering in living cells. Proc Natl Acad Sci USA 2008; 105:7405-9.
6. Phizicky E, Fields S. Protein-protein interactions: methods for detection and analysis. Microbiol Rev 1995; 59:94-123.
7. Van Criekinge W, Beyaert R. Yeast two-hybrid: state of the art. biol proced online (www.biologicalprocedures.com) 1999; 2:1-38.
8. Niethammer M, Sheng M. Identification of ion channel-associated proteins using the yeast two-hybrid system. Methods Enzymol 1998; 293:104-22.
9. Guo D, Rajamäki ML, Valkonen. Protein-protein interactions: the yeast two hybrid system. Methods Mol Biol 2008; 451:421-39.
10. Larkin D, Murphy D, Reilly DF et al. ICln, a novel integrin alpha(IIb)beta3-associated protein, functionally regulates platelet activation. J Biol Chem 2004; 279:27286-93.
11. Lal A, Haynes SR, Gorospe M. Clean western blot signals from immunoprecipitated samples. Mol Cell Probe 2005; 19:385-8.
12. Ransone LJ. Detection of protein protein interactions by coimmunoprecipitation and dimerization. Method Enzymol 1995; 254:491-7.
13. Qoronfleh MW, Ren L, Emery D et al. Use of immunomatrix methods to improve protein-protein interaction detection, J Biomed Biotechnol 2003; 2003(5):291-8.
14. McPhee JC, Dang YL, Davidson N et al. Evidence for a functional interaction between integrins and G protein-activated inward rectifier K$^+$ channels. J Biol Chem 1998; 273; 34696-702.
15. Ivanina T, Neusch C, Yong-Xin L et al. Expression of GIRK (Kir3.1/Kir3.4) channels in mouse fibroblast cells with and without β1 integrins. FEBS Letts 2000; 466:327-32.
16. Levite M, Cahalon L, Peretz A et al. Extracellular K$^+$ and opening of voltage-gated potassium channels activate T-cell integrin function: physical and functional association between Kv1.3 channels and beta1 integrins. J Exp Med 2000; 191:1167-76.
17. Alessandri Haber N, Olayinka AD, Joseph EK et al. Interaction of transient receptor potential vanilloid 4, integrin and SRC tyrosine kinase in mechanical hyperalgesia. J Neurosci 2008; 28:1046-57.
18. Cherubini A, Pillozzi S, Hofmann G et al. HERG K$^+$ channels and β1 integrins interact through the assembly of a macromolecular complex. Ann NY Acad Sci 2002; 973:559-61.
19. Cherubini A, Hofmann G, Pillozzi S et al. Herg1 channels are physically linked to beta 1 integrins and modulate adhesion-dependent signalling. Mol Biol Cell 2005; 16:2972-83.
20. Abdel-Ghany M, Cheng HC, Elble RC et al. The interacting binding domains of the beta4 integrin and calcium-activated chloride channels (CLCAs) in metastasis. J Biol Chem 2003; 278:49406-16.
21. Wyszynski M, Sheng M. Analysis of ion channels associated proteins. Methods Enzymol 1999; 294:371-385.
22. Nooren IMA, Thornten MA. J Mol Biol 2003; 325:991-1018.
23. Bomgarden RD. Studying protein interactions in living cells. Genetic Engineering and Biotechnology News (www.genengnews.com) 2008; 28(7).
24. Fancy D. Elucidation of protein-protein interactions using chemical cross-linking or label transfer techniques. Curr Opin Chem Biol 2000; 4:28-33.
25. Häse CC, Minchin RF, Kloda A et al. Cross-linking studies and membrane localization and assembly of radiolabelled large mechanosensitive ion channel (MscL) of Escherichia coli. Biochem Biophys Res Comm 1997; 232:777-82.
26. Mahlknecht U, Ottmann OG, Hoelzer D. J Biotechnol 2001; 88:89-94.

27. Abdel-Ghany M, Cheng HC, Elble RC et al. The breast cancer β4 integrin and endothelial human CLCA2 mediate lung metastasis. J Biol Chem 2001; 276:25438-46.
28. Howell JM, Winstone TL, Coorssen JR et al. An evaluation of in vitro protein-protein interaction techniques: assessing contaminating background proteins. Proteomics 2006; 6:2050-69.
29. Arcangeli A, Becchetti A, Mannini A et al. Integrin-mediated neurite outgrowth in neuroblastoma cells depends on the activation of potassium channels. J Cell Biol 1993; 122:1131-43.
30. Davis MJ, Wu X, Nurkiewicz TR et al. Regulation of ion channels by integrins. Cell Biochem Biophys 2002; 36:41-66.
31. Hofmann G, Bernabei PA, Crociani O et al. HERG K+ channels activation during β1 Integrin-mediated Adhesion to fibronectin induces an up-regulation of αvβ3 Integrin in the preosteoclastic leukemia cell line FLG 29.1. J Biol Chem 2001; 276:4923-31.
32. Waitkus-Edwards KR, Martinez-Lemus LA, Trzeciakovski JP et al. α4β1 integrin activation of L-type calcium channels in vascular smooth muscle causes arteriole vasoconstriction. Circ Res 2002; 90:473-80.
33. Yang W, Steen H, Freeman MR. Proteomic approaches to the analysis of multiprotein signalling complexes. Proteomics 2008; 8:832-51.
34. Bunnell SC, Hong DI, Kardon JR et al. T-cell receptor ligation induces the formation of dynamically regulated signaling assemblies. J Cell Biol 2002; 58:1263-1275.

Chapter 4

Optical Methods in the Study of Protein-Protein Interactions

Alessio Masi, Riccardo Cicchi, Adolfo Carloni, Francesco Saverio Pavone and Annarosa Arcangeli*

Abstract

Förster (or Fluorescence) resonance energy transfer (FRET) is a physical process in which energy is transferred nonradiatively from an excited fluorophore, serving as a donor, to another chromophore (acceptor). Among the techniques related to fluorescence microscopy, FRET is unique in providing signals sensitive to intra- and intermolecular distances in the 1-10 nm range. Because of its potency, FRET is increasingly used to visualize and quantify the dynamics of protein-protein interaction in living cells, with high spatio-temporal resolution.

Here we describe the physical bases of FRET, detailing the principal methods applied: (1) measurement of signal intensity and (2) analysis of fluorescence lifetime (FLIM). Although several technical complications must be carefully considered, both methods can be applied fruitfully to specific fields. For example, FRET based on intensity detection is more suitable to follow biological phenomena at a finely tuned spatial and temporal scale. Furthermore, a specific fluorescence signal occurring close to the plasma membrane (≤100 nm) can be obtained using a total internal reflection fluorescence (TIRF) microscopy system.

When performing FRET experiments, care must be also taken to the method chosen for labeling interacting proteins. Two principal tools can be applied: (1) fluorophore tagged antibodies; (2) recombinant fluorescent fusion proteins. The latter method essentially takes advantage of the discovery and use of spontaneously fluorescent proteins, like the green fluorescent protein (GFP).

Until now, FRET has been widely used to analyze the structural characteristics of several proteins, including integrins and ion channels. More recently, this method has been applied to clarify the interaction dynamics of these classes of membrane proteins with cytosolic signaling proteins.

We report two examples in which the interaction dynamics between integrins and ion channels have been studied with FRET methods. Using fluorescent antibodies and applying FRET-FLIM, the direct interaction of β1 integrin with the receptor for Epidermal Growth Factor (EGF-R) has been proved in living endothelial cells. A different approach, based on TIRFM measurement of the FRET intensity of fluorescently labeled recombinant proteins, suggests that a direct interaction also occurs between integrins and the ether-à-go-go-related-gene 1 (hERG1) K+ channel.

*Corresponding Author: Annarosa Arcangeli—Department of Experimental Pathology and Oncology, University of Firenze. Viale G.B. Morgagni 50, 50134 Firenze-Italy. Email: annarosa.arcangeli@unifi.it

Integrins and Ion Channels: Molecular Complexes and Signaling, edited by Andrea Becchetti and Annarosa Arcangeli. ©2010 Landes Bioscience and Springer Science+Business Media.

Introduction

Most physiological processes are based on physicochemical phenomena such as molecular binding, association, conformational changes etc. Structural hierarchies inside mammalian cells, supracellular organization in tissues as well as communication at both the cell and tissue levels are imposed through a network of cascade and feedback mechanisms based on the above reactions. Hence, a full elucidation of biological processes requires thorough study of the spatio-temporal distribution and the functional states of the constituent molecules. Besides localization of proteins with imaging methods, monitoring of their interaction and function is a prerequisite to understand their cellular role. From this standpoint, fluorescence microscopy is an ideal method, since it can generate the necessary level of optical contrast by exploiting different manifestations of light emission, to obtain the required sensitivity, selectivity and modulation via reactions in the ground and excited electronic states. In this way, it is possible to produce a well defined map of intracellular and plasmamembrane molecules as well as their reciprocal interactions. In the past two decades, fluorescence microscopy has greatly benefited from the introduction of new chemical and molecular tools that, in combination with the advancements in laser microscopy and photo-detection technologies, have considerably expanded its applications. Especially relevant to life science research has been the advent of new biological probes, such as labeled antibodies and fluorescent recombinant proteins. These now permit to attain high specificity and resolution in imaging biological molecules, especially proteins. Fluorescent antibodies allow to detect and map the expression of a given protein within a single cell, a cellular monolayer or a tissue section. The sole limitation of this approach is the availability of good antibodies. Moreover, a new era in protein imaging has been started by the discovery of spontaneously fluorescent proteins coupled with DNA manipulation techniques.[1,2] The Green Fluorescent Protein (GFP) from the jellyfish *Aequoria Victoria* was the first such protein to be found and it is still the best characterized. It is in fact a genetically encoded fluorophore, which means that the GFP coding sequence can be fused with that of any other gene to give a fused fluorescent protein that can be localized inside a living cell.

The availability of such techniques has given life scientists the power to label and image virtually any protein in any cell line or tissue or even in living organisms, with an especially strong impact for the study of protein-protein interactions. By labeling the target proteins, it is possible to take advantage of the spectral interactions between fluorophores, in order to obtain spatial and functional information about protein interactions. Quenching, for example, is the darkening of a fluorophore's emission due to the transfer of energy, in a nonradiative fashion, to a molecule standing in close vicinity (~10 nm), called quencher. In this process, the excited fluorophore relaxes without the emission of a photon. However, if the quencher is a fluorescent molecule as well, it relaxes by re-emitting a photon. This phenomenon is known as Förster (or Flourescence) Resonance Energy Transfer (FRET).

Förster Resonance Energy Transfer: The "Molecular Ruler"

FRET, originally described by Theodor Förster in 1948,[3] is a radiationless transfer of energy from an excited fluorophore (named donor) to a nearby fluorophore (named acceptor). The acceptor undergoes a transition to an excited state rapidly followed by the emission of a photon. The emitted photon is always at a longer wavelength (lower energy) compared to that absorbed by the donor. For the process to occur, the donor and acceptor molecules, called a FRET pair, must meet the following requirements (see also Fig. 1A): (1) the emission spectrum of the donor must overlap significantly with the absorption spectrum of the acceptor and (2) the two molecules must be in close vicinity (5-10 nm), since the efficiency of this interaction is inversely related to the 6th power of the inter-molecular distance. In fact

$$E = [1 + (r/R_0)^6]^{-1}$$

where E is the efficiency, r is the intermolecular distance and R_0, known as Förster constant, is the value of r where FRET efficiency is 50%. Depending on the fluorophore pair, this value

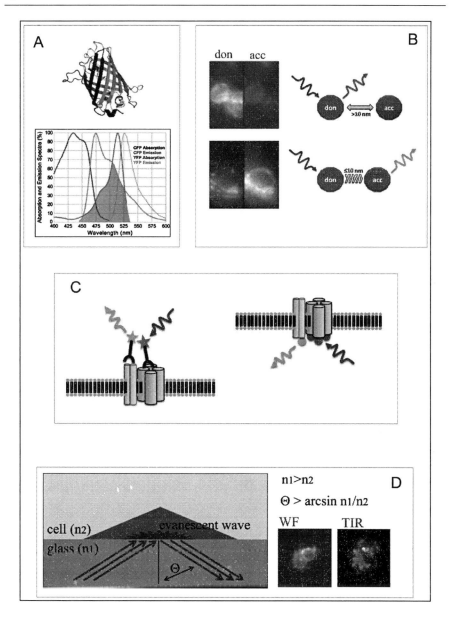

Figure 1. Biological applications of FRET and TIRFM. A) Top: Crystal structure of the Green Fluorescent Protein. Bottom: Spectral properties of GFP-related CFP and YFP, a commonly used FRET pair (courtesy of Ormo M et al.(1996) Crystal structure of the Aequorea victoria green fluorescent protein. Science 273: 1392-1395). B) microphotographs showing the shift in signal intensity, imaged with a CCD, upon protein interaction. Images were obtained by the authors in HEK 293 cells transfected with HERG-CFP and β1 integrin-YFP (unpublished). C) Antibody- (left) versus fusion protein- (right) based detection of membrane protein interaction with FRET. The cartoon shows an integrin dimer interacting with an ion channel. D) Schematic representation of the TIR principle (left). The two microphotographs show the difference in resolution and spatial information when exciting the same cell in wide field (WF) mode versus TIR. A color version of this image is available at www.landesbioscience.com/curie.

ranges from 2 to 8 nm. If these conditions are satisfied, the donor's emission is quenched and the acceptor's emission is intensified (sensitised) proportionally. As a result of the strong dependence of FRET efficiency on the intermolecular distance between the two interplaying molecules, a major experimental application to life science is the potential to determine intra- and inter-molecular distances in the 1-10 nm range, hence the nickname, whether at steady-state or in dynamic conditions. In other words, FRET is capable of resolving molecular interactions and conformations with a spatial resolution far exceeding the inherent diffraction limit ($\sim\lambda/2$) of conventional optical microscopy, yet is also compatible with super-resolution techniques.

Experimentally, FRET can be detected and estimated mainly in two ways: by quantifying the energy being transferred in the process (in terms of donor quenching or acceptor sensitisation), or by measuring donor fluorescence lifetime.

Intensity Versus Lifetime: Two Ways to Measure FRET

Regardless of the method chosen to label interacting proteins (see below), two different parameters can be measured when attempting to detect FRET signals arising from interacting proteins: (1) signal intensity and (2) fluorescence lifetime.

Detection of signal intensity was the first to be developed. Briefly, during sample illumination, emission from the two fluorophores is split, filtered through a specific filter set and collected separately by one or two detectors, i.e., a photomultiplier or a CCD camera. The intensity of donor and acceptor signals are compared and FRET is detected as an intensification in the acceptor's emission, or as a synchronous decrease in donor's emission. This method allows to acquire image frames for the entire duration of the biological process under study. Furthermore, time-lapse imaging can help reduce photobleaching, especially of the donor. This method, very simple and straightforward in principle, is biased by some complications, that must be taken into account before planning or accomplishing any FRET experiment. First, spectral overlap must always be taken into consideration. The wavelength at which the donor is excited can in turn excite to some extent the acceptor itself, resulting in a fluorescent signal from the acceptor. As a consequence, if the acceptor concentration in the biological sample is significantly higher than the donor's, the signal from the acceptor may turn out to be more intense than the one from the donor, even in the absence of energy transfer. This can be misinterpreted as a FRET signal. Second, the donor's emission always leaks in the acceptor channel, which needs to be carefully estimated and factored out. Other phenomena, such as saturation or bleaching, can bias FRET measurements in a poorly predictable manner. Donor bleaching, for example, will inevitably occur and be faster than bleaching of the acceptor, as the donor must be excited in order to have FRET and this leads to errors in calculating FRET efficiency.

The second technique, Fluorescence Lifetime Imaging Microscopy (FLIM) has the remarkable advantage of being independent from intensity, as fluorophore interaction is detected in terms of variations of fluorescence lifetime (shortening, in the case of the donor's emission).[4] Experimentally, lifetime imaging is achieved by (1) measuring the latency between the absorption of an excitation photon and the emission of a fluorescent photon by the donor (Time-Domain FLIM), or (2) the phase-shift in emission frequency compared to excitation frequency (Frequency-Domain FLIM). In either case, a pulsed excitation source is required. Lifetime variations are due to intra- and inter-molecular factors. The former are usually probe-specific, whereas the latter are related to the chemical or biological micro-environment. In this respect, FRET results in a measurable shortening of donor's lifetime, since dipole-dipole interactions accelerate the non radiative relaxation phase and thus photon emission.

Understandably, most of the issues affecting intensity-based FRET are of no concern in FLIM, with the notable exception of spectra overlap, which must be taken into account in FLIM too. On the other hand, due to the low excitation intensity required, FLIM has relatively long acquisition times (30 seconds or more) and thus the time resolution is relatively poor, making this technique unsuited to the detection of fast events (see Fig. 2).

Optical Methods in the Study of Protein-Protein Interactions

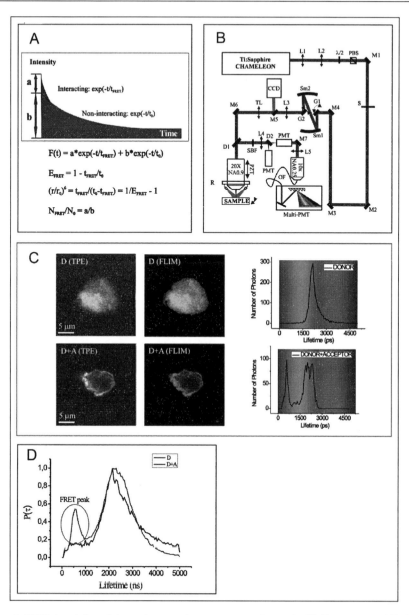

Figure 2. FRET signals from interacting membrane receptors imaged with Fluorescence Lifetime Microscopy. A) Principles of FRET-FLIM and equations used to calculate lifetimes and FRET efficiency. B) Schematic depiction of the nonlinear microscope used in FLIM-FRET experiments. C) Two-photon fluorescence image of a cell acquired using single photon counting technique (TPE, left) and the corresponding FLIM pseudo-color image (middle), obtained after system-response de-convolution and single-exponential fit. The color-scale is shown in graph (right), together with the lifetime distribution of image pixels. Upper row refers to control situation where only the donor (D) antibody is present. Lower row refers to FRET conditions where both donor and acceptor (D + A) are present. D) Averaged mean lifetime distribution of cells labelled with: donor alone, donor + acceptor. A color version of this image is available at www.landesbioscience.com/curie.

Total Internal Reflection Fluorescence Microscopy (TIRFM) and Imaging of Membrane Proteins

A major disadvantage of applying FRET to living cells is interference of signals not related to the interaction of the two molecules under study. An example is cellular autofluorescence, which can be excluded by confining the excitation signal to a minute volume, containing the molecule of interest. This can be realized either by confocal or Total Internal Reflection Fluorescence (TIRF) microscopy. For the observation of many types of live cells, relatively large areas need often to be imaged at high resolution, in a short time. If confocal microscopy is employed for this task, the time to acquire sufficient signals per pixel puts a limit to the total imaging times. In contrast, as TIRFM does not suffer from this limitation and represents a powerful alternative for imaging large areas. Furthermore, TIRFM can be applied in conjunction with FRET to detect dynamic informations from membrane proteins. Hence, coupling TIRFM with FRET is becoming one of the preferred methods to follow the interaction between plasma membrane proteins.

TIRFM is an optical phenomenon whereby an incident light beam, propagating through a medium 1 of refractive index n_1 (i.e., a glass slide) encounters a medium 2 of refractive index $n_2 < n_1$ (i.e., the cytoplasm) with an angle σ bigger than the critical angle σ (defined as arcsin n_2/n_1). The incident beam is thus totally reflected and generates, in medium 2, a so-called evanescent wave that decays with the 6th power of the distance, hence within ~300 nm. If a fluorescent molecule is located within 300 nm from the glass surface and the reflected beam has the right wavelength and intensity, this molecule will fluoresce yielding information on this very thin section that corresponds, in our example, to the cell-substrate interface (Fig. 1D; for a review on biological applications of TIRFM see ref. 5).

Antibody-Based Versus Fusion Protein-Based FRET: Principles

As mentioned above, to study the spatial localization and interaction of two protein types (hereafter referred to as A and B), the target protein must be fluorescently labeled in order to obtain a FRET signal. The FRET fluorophore pair must meet the requirements discussed in the previous section and, depending on its molecular structure, specific labeling procedures can be applied. Let us consider a hypothetical experiment, in which the researcher wants to determine whether two different membrane proteins are physically associated in basal conditions, or become associated upon exposure to a certain stimulus. After gathering results with more typical biochemical approaches, such as co-immunoprecipitation and thus finding that A an B might be part of a molecular complex, the researcher can seek independent confirmation with a radically different approach, such as FRET. If specific antibodies, preferably monoclonal, for A and B are available, one possibility is labeling the antibody pair with proper fluorophores. As discussed earlier, the ideal donor should have an emission spectrum that fully overlaps with the absorption spectrum of the acceptor, whereas the two excitation spectra should be totally separated. In practice, neither condition is ever fully met and exciting the donor molecule usually produces some degree of acceptor excitation as well. A number of commercially available labeling kits permit to conjugate many different fluorescent molecules to virtually any antibody. To obtain covalent binding, dyes are modified by the addition of chemical groups, usually esters, that react with amino residues, to form amide bonds. Conjugated antibodies are then purified through an affinity-column. After purification, the degree of labeling of the antibodies is estimated by measuring the absorbance at 280 nm, the protein absorption wavelength, and at the dye's specific wavelength. The conjugated antibodies can then be used in any of the numerous immuno-fluorescence procedures described in the literature. The sample under investigation, a cell line for example, can be processed for detection of FRET signal. In this case, cells are fixed and then incubated with a blocking solution (normally bovine serum albumin, in standard saline solution). Subsequently, they are incubated with the labeled antibodies and mounted on a microscope slide. Alternatively, normal primary IgGs can be used followed by incubation with commercial conjugated anti-IgG antibodies. As a general rule, use of labeled primary antibodies provides highest specificity, whereas use of labeled secondaries gives brighter signal.

The procedure described so forth only yields information about the state of the investigated proteins at the time when cells are fixed. If one is interested in the dynamics of the process, which is known or hypothesized to be transient or cyclic, this approach is useless. One way to overcome this limitation, is to use the fluorescent antibody set directly on living cells, so that the biological process involving the interaction between A and B can be triggered at will and monitored in real-time. This is easier in the case of plasma membrane proteins, but it is also possible when studying cytosolic proteins, as the injection and function of antibodies in living cells has been described.[6] The time-course of the process under investigation can then be monitored by acquiring images from single cells regularly challenged with proper excitation pulses. The cellular localization of A and B can be screened over time thanks to fluorescence. Their physical association, when occurring, can be detected from assembling to disassembling by following the kinetics of the FRET signal.

The second approach to FRET-based protein-protein interaction study depends on the production of fused genes, as permitted by the modern cloning techniques, now routinely carried out in most laboratories. Such genes can be introduced in living cells and normally transcribed and translated to generate functional proteins. In our hypothetical experiment, the genes encoding A and B could be cloned and fused for example with Cyan Fluorescent Protein (CFP, a blue-shifted mutant of GFP) and Yellow Fluorescent Protein (YFP, a red-shifted mutant of GFP) respectively. The two fusion genes could be then introduced into a suitable expression vector, to generate a transgenic cell line expressing, constitutively or upon induction, both A-CFP and B-YFP. If necessary, stable transfectants can be selected and clones produced that display the desired expression levels of the two proteins. Subsequently, optical methods analogous to those outlined above are applied to the genetically modified cells. Therefore, both methods converge after proteins have been labeled. However, the two approaches present both biological and optical issues that make them different and not always interchangeable.

Antibody-Based Versus Fusion Protein-Based FRET: Advantages and Disadvantages

Antibody-based FRET has the remarkable advantage that it can be used to image endogenous proteins. In other words, this method allows to study wild type cells, whereas the fusion protein-based FRET needs genetic manipulation, which can perturbate the cellular physiology. Fusion proteins may in fact show significantly altered function, structure or lifetime. Hence, careful (sometimes troublesome!) characterisation is recommended prior to experiment execution. In addition, endogenous wild-type A and B may be expressed by the engineered cell and this implies the assumption that exogenous and endogenous proteins act in a similar way, so that the data obtained with the fusion proteins A and B are representative of the endogenous homologues. Finally, careful consideration must be devoted to fusion protein design, as fluorescent appendages can be attached indifferently to either termini (N- or C-) of proteins. However, if CFP and YFP are too far apart, no FRET signal will be detected, even if A and B are physically associated.

In spite of these considerations, a fusion protein-based approach is generally preferred, because of the shortcomings of the antibody-based method. Antibody binding often presents insufficient specificity and efficiency, especially in living cells, where blocking may not be possible. In addition, antigens, i.e., A and B, may be hidden or not efficiently accessible to labeled antibodies. Even when they are, only an indirect estimate about the protein-protein distance is given, as FRET occurs between fluorophore residues that are attached in variable positions on the antibodies, thus reducing the accuracy of the measure. Overall, these factors often lead to poor specificity, high background fluorescence and a reduction in signal-to-noise ratio. In contrast, fusion proteins provide higher specificity and lower background, as fluorescence signal comes exclusively from CFP and YFP moieties. Moreover, because each A is bound to one CFP and each B is bound to one YFP, the labeling is 1:1. This greatly simplifies the calculations of FRET efficiency and the quantification of protein interactions (Fig. 1B,C).

Application of Optical Methods to the Study of Integrins and Ion Channels

For the reasons discussed earlier, the literature on protein-protein interaction and FRET offers numerous examples of fusion protein-based measurements, but much fewer antibody-based studies. The CFP/YFP couple is indeed the most common FRET pair employed for creating such fusion proteins. Considering the object of the present book, we will briefly review the studies focused on integrins and ion channels. Almost all of the techniques outlined above have been used to define both conformational features and molecular dynamics of these membrane proteins.

Several studies have focused on structural characteristics. For example Coutinho and coworkers[7] tested by FRET the proposed structural rearrangements undergone by integrin β_3 after cell activation. They attached fluorescent labels to Fab fragments of monoclonal antibodies directed to the βA domain of the β_3 subunit and to the Calf-2 domain of the α_{IIb} subunit. The data thus obtained in living cells were consistent with a conformational model of the activated integrin less extended than in the switchblade model previously proposed. Nevertheless, the major application of FRET has been to analyze integrin signaling. A recent survey on this topic reported the development of genetically encoded and FRET-based biosensors for imaging the integrin-related signaling cascade.[8] In particular, a FRET biosensor for Src kinase has provided a complementary approach to the traditional biochemical assays for studying integrin function and association with other signaling molecules. The time-resolution and subcellular visualization enabled by different FRET approaches has shed new light on the molecular mechanisms regulating integrin signaling. A novel application of FRET-FLIM to integrins has been recently utilized by the Humphries' research group to address the still unsolved question of the integrin-effector binding and the response of these interactions to antagonists.[9] Employing integrin-GFP and effector-Red Fluorescent Protein (-RFP) pairs in living cells and quantifying their association using FLIM to measure FRET, revealed an unexpected agonistic activity of small molecules (RGD and LDV mimetics), classically used as integrin inhibitors.

Other studies, mainly employing the CFP/YFP FRET pair and labeled recombinant proteins, have greatly contributed to uncover the molecular architecture of ion channels, both ligand-[10,11] and voltage-gated. In the former, application of FRET has also contributed to unravel the conformational rearrangements associated with ligand binding.[12] In voltage-gated ion channels, great insight about the conformational changes that accompany the gating process has been offered by FRET.[13,14] The analysis of heterotetramer assembly in voltage dependent K$^+$ channels has also greatly benefited from the FRET technique. When applied to Kv 1.3 and Kv 1.5, FRET analysis confirmed the existence of functional hybrid channels as well as their colocalization into caveolae.[15] In an interesting paper by Maurel and coworkers,[16] the hetero-dimerisation of the B1 and B2 subunits of the γ-amino-butyric acid (GABA) receptor, which is induced by GABA administration, is used as a model system to implement a method for immuno-detection of FRET events. HEK 293 cells were transfected with haemagglutin GABA$_{B1}$ and myc epitope-tagged GABA$_{B2}$. Antibodies against either tag were labelled with Eu-cryptate-PBP and Alexa 647 respectively. FRET was then triggered by GABA application and detected with a dual-wavelength single-cell fluorimeter. FRET has also been applied to detect ligand-induced conformational changes in the cytoplasmic domains of ligand-gated ion channels, a topic particularly difficult to solve exclusively with a biochemical approach.[17] Finally, ion channel binding to different signaling proteins has been also studied with FRET. For example, Shapiro and collaborators carried out FRET-TIRFM studies to determine direct interaction between CFP-tagged KCNQ2-4 channels and YFP-tagged calmodulin, both expressed in CHO cells.[18] A recent paper using a similar approach reported that the actin binding protein cortactin regulates the potassium channel Kv 1.2, since the two proteins directly interact in vivo.[19] These results prove that a direct link occurs between actin dynamics and membrane excitability.

FLIM has also recently been used in our laboratories to investigate the EGFR- β1 integrin interaction induced by β1 integrin stimulation in living endothelial cells.[20] ECV 304 cells were first incubated with Alexa 488 anti-EGFR alone, then with Alexa 546 TS2/16, an activating anti-β1 antibody known to trigger the formation of the EGFR-integrin membrane complex. Using FLIM, FRET was detected in a reproducible and controlled way. Measures obtained in cells treated as described above showed that (1) FRET occurs between fluorescently labeled EGFR and activated integrin receptors, (2) this process is Src kinase-dependent and (3) the process is enhanced in presence of EGF.

What about the possibility of detecting ion channel/integrin interactions by applying the FRET technique? Until now, the only evidence about this issue is provided by the work of Artym and Petty (2002), who used direct and indirect immunolabeling of β1 integrin and $K_v1.3$ channels, in paraformaldehyde-fixed cell lines. In this work, the FRET pair used was FIT-C/TRIT-C. Energy transfer was measured by detecting fluorescence intensity with both a CCD camera and single cell spectrometry. Results showed that $β_1$ integrin and $K_v1.3$ present close proximity and that this association occurs in adhesion-dependent manner.[21]

Recently FRET experiments performed in our laboratory, confirmed the direct interaction between β1 integrin and hERG1 channels previously suggested by biochemical methods.[22] As fully described in Chapter 6, this result was obtained using recombinant fluorescent proteins, YFP-integrin and CFP-hERG1, transfected into HEK 293 cells. Images were analyzed with a TIRFM apparatus, to detect only the proteins expressed onto the plasma membrane.

Conclusion

FRET is unique in generating fluorescence signals sensitive to molecular conformation, association and separation, in the 1-10 nm range. Hence, it is the technique of choice when studying the molecular dynamics of proteins especially in the context of protein-protein interactions. When coupled with TIRM, this method can be applied to detect protein dynamics at the plasma membrane level.

FRET has been successfully applied to the study of the structure of adhesion receptors and ion channels, in living cells and organisms. Moreover, it is now greatly contributing to define the molecular interactions between these types of membrane proteins. Once the functional link between a specific integrin and an ion channel type is determined, the subsequent step is studying whether these proteins form complexes on the plasma membrane, possibly with the partecipation of other proteins. To this purpose, the biochemical methods outlined in the previous chapter are invaluable. However, once the occurrence of a complex has been defined in this way, further analysis with FRET-based methods provide the most unequivocal conclusions about the occurrence of the complex and its molecular structure and functional dynamics.

To date, a lot has been done to tune the methodological aspects of the technique. Time has now come to apply these ever more specialized and sophisticated techniques to address fundamental biological questions, such as the mechanisms underlying inter- and intracellular communications.

Acknowledgements

This work has been supported by grants from the Associazione Italiana per la Ricerca sul Cancro (AIRC), the Association for International Cancer Research (AICR), the Ministero dell'Università e della Ricerca Scientifica e Tecnologica (PRIN 2005), the Associazione Genitori Noi per Voi, the Ente Cassa di Risparmio di Firenze (to AA) and the Ente Cassa di Risparmio di Firenze (to FSP).

References

1. Prasher DC, Eckenrode VK, Ward WW et al. Primary structure of the aequorea victoria green-fluorescent protein. Gene 1992; 111:229-33.
2. Ormo M, Cubitt AB, Kallio K et al. Crystal structure of the aequorea victoria green fluorescent protein. Science 1996; 273:1392-1395.
3. Förster T. Zwischenmolekulare energiewanderung und fluoreszenz. Ann Physik 1948; 437:55-61.
4. Lakowicz JR, Szmacinski H, Nowaczyk K et al. Fluorescence lifetime imaging of free and protein-bound NADH. Proc Natl Acad Sci USA 1992; 89:1271-1275.
5. Schneckenburger H. Total internal reflection fluorescence microscopy: technical innovations and novel applications. Curr Opin Biotechnol 2005; 16:13-18.

6. Morgan DO, Roth RA. Analysis of intracellular protein function by antibody injection. Immunol Today 1988; 9:84-98.
7. Coutinho A, Garcia C, Gonzalez-Rodriguez J et al. Conformational changes in human $\alpha_{IIb}\beta_3$ after platelet activation, monitored by FRET. Biophys Chem 2007; 130:76-87.
8. Wang Y, Chien S. Analysis of integrin signaling by fluorescence resonance energy transfer. Methods in Enzymol 2007; 426:177-201.
9. Parsons M, Messent AJ, Humphries JD et al. Quantification of integrin receptor agonism by fluorescence lifetime imaging. J Cell Sci 2007; 121:265-271.
10. Oung MT, Fisher JA, Fountain SJ et al. Molecular shape, architecture and size of P2X4 receptors determined using fluorescence resonance energy transfer and electron microscopy. J Biol Chem 2008; pub online.
11. Nashmi R, Dickinson ME, McKinney S et al. Assembly of alpha4beta2 nicotinic acetylcholine receptors assessed with functional fluorescently labelled subunits: effects of localization, trafficking and nicotine-induced upregulation in clonal mammalian cells and in cultured midbrain neurons. J Neurosci 2003; 23:11554-11567.
12. Taraska JW, Zagotta WN. Structural dynamics in the gating ring of cyclic nucleotide-gated ion channels. Nat Struct Mol Biol 2007; 14:854-860.
13. Kobrinsky E, Stevens L, Kazmi Y et al. Molecular rearrangements of the Kv2.1 potassium channel termini associated with voltage gating. J Biol Chem 2006; 281:19233-19240.
14. Riven I, Kalmanzon E, Segev L et al. Conformational rearrangements associated with the gating of the G protein-coupled potassium channel revealed by FRET microscopy. Neuron 2003; 38:225-235.
15. Vicente R, Villalonga N, Calvo M et al. Kv 1.5 association modifies Kv 1.3 traffic and membrane localization. J Biol Chem 2008; 283:8756-8764.
16. Maurel D, Kniazeff J, Mathis G et al. Cell surface detection of membrane protein interaction with homogeneous time-resolved fluorescence resonance energy transfer technology. Anal Biochem 2004; 329:253-262.
17. Tateyama M, Abe H, Nakata H et al. Ligand-induced rearrangements of the dimeric metabotropic glutamate receptor 1α. Nature Struct Mol Biol 2004; 11:637-642.
18. Bal M, Zaika O, Martin P et al. Calmodulin binding to M-type K⁺ channels assayed by TIRF/FRET in living cells. J Physiol 2008; 586:2307-2320.
19. Williams MR, Markey JC, Doczi MA et al. As essential role for cortactin in the modulation of the potassium channel Kv 1.2. Proc Natl Acad Sci USA 2007; 104:17412-17417.
20. Cabodi S, Morello V, Masi A et al. Convergence of integrins and EGF receptor signaling via PI3K/Akt/FoxO pathway in early gene Egr-1 transcription. J Cell Physiol 2009; 218: 294-303
21. Artym VV, Petty HR. Molecular proximity of Kv1.3 Voltage-gated potassium channels and integrins on the plasma membrane of melanoma cells: effects of cell adherence and channel blockers. J Gen Physiol 2002; 120:29-37.
22. Cherubini A, Hofmann G, Pillozzi S et al. hERG1 channels are physically linked to beta1 integrins and modulate adhesion-dependent signalling. Mol Biol Cell 2005; 16:2972-2983.

CHAPTER 5

Integrins and Signal Transduction

Sara Cabodi, Paola Di Stefano, Maria del Pilar Camacho Leal, Agata Tinnirello, Brigitte Bisaro, Virginia Morello, Laura Damiano, Simona Aramu, Daniele Repetto, Giusy Tornillo and Paola Defilippi*

Abstract

Integrin signaling has a critical function in organizing cells in tissues during both embryonic development and tissue repair. Following their binding to the extracellular ligands, the intracellular signaling pathways triggered by integrins are directed to two major functions: organization of the actin cytoskeleton and regulation of cell behaviour including survival, differentiation and growth. Basic research conducted in the past twelve years has lead to remarkable breakthroughs in this field. Integrins are catalytically inactive and translate positional cues into biochemical signals by direct and/or functional association with intracellular adaptors, cytosolic tyrosine kinases or growth factor and cytokine receptors. The purpose of this chapter is to highlight recent experimental and conceptual advances in integrin signaling with particular emphasis on the ability of integrins to regulate Fak/Src family kinases (SFKs) activation and the cross-talk with soluble growth factors receptors and cytokines.

Overview of Integrin Structure

Structural Features of the Integrin Family

Integrins are cell surface heterodimeric receptors formed by the non covalent association of α and β subunits. The mammalian genome comprises 8 β subunit and 18 α subunit genes, that assemble into 24 different functional integrins (Table 1).[1] Integrins are transmembrane proteins characterised by a large extracellular domain that forms elongated stalks and a globular ligand-binding head regions and a short cytoplasmic tails connected to the actin cytoskeleton. Most β subunits contain in their cytoplasmic region a NPxY sequence which can associate to cytoskeletal and signaling proteins that contain a phosphotyrosine binding (PTB) domain. In addition, alternative splicing regions in the extracellular and cytoplasmic domains give rise to variant forms of both α and β subunits.

On the basis of integrin binding to components of the extracellular matrix such as collagen, laminin and RGD receptors, integrins can be ascribed to different subfamilies. While common integrin binding domain represented by the short peptide RGD (Arg-Gly-Asp) is present on fibronectin, vitronectin and fibrinogen, laminin and collagens contain different binding domains. In addition, integrins expressed on the hematopoietic compartment bind to counter receptors such as VCAM or ICAM-1 (Table 1).

Connection between the ECM and the Actin Cytoskeleton

Integrins specifically localize to focal adhesions, which are sites of close apposition with the extracellular matrix (ECM) where actin filament are anchored to the plasma membrane.[2] At these sites,

*Corresponding Author: Paola Defilippi—Molecular and Biotechnology Center and Department of Genetics, Biology and Biochemistry, University of Torino, Via Nizza 52, 10126, Torino, Italy. Email: paola.defilippi@unito.it

Integrins and Ion Channels: Molecular Complexes and Signaling, edited by Andrea Becchetti and Annarosa Arcangeli. ©2010 Landes Bioscience and Springer Science+Business Media.

Table 1. Integrin heterodimers and substrate binding

Type of Integrin Receptor		Substrates
α Subunit	β Subunit	
α1	β1	Collagen
α2		
α9		
α10		
α11		
α7	β1	Laminin
α3	β1	
α6	β1, β4	
α5	β1	RGD
αv	β1, β3	
α8	β1	
αIIb2	β3	
α4	β1	
α4	β7	VCAM
αE	β7	E-Cadherin
αL, αd	β2	ICAM, VCAM
αM, αX	β2	Fibrinogen

integrins codistribute with cytoskeletal proteins such as talin, kindlin, vinculin and α actinin, which are prominent integrin-associated structural proteins which bind F-actin, thus recruiting actin filaments to integrin clusters. In addition, these integrin-associated molecules serve as multi-functional scaffolding proteins, leading to protein-protein interactions by the recruitment of kinases, phophatases and their substrates together, thus regulating the dynamic of integrin-cytoskeleton connection (Fig. 1).[3]

Integrin activation results from the ability to assume various affinity states that can be regulated bidirectionally either by "outside in" signaling, induced by cell-ECM interaction, or "inside-out signaling", where intracellular events involving the cytoplasmic domains of α and β integrin subunits are coupled to extracellular conformational changes induced by extracellular factors.[4] Thus, integrins can move from an inactive state, in which they do not bind ligands, to an active state, in which they behave as high affinity receptors (Fig. 2). Integrin activation is mainly regulated by talin, a large major actin-binding protein which associate to the cytoplasmic domain of β subunits with its FERM (Four-point-one, Ezrin, Radixin, Moesin) domain. Talin binding to integrins disrupts an intracellular salt bridge between the α and the β subunit, leading to increased integrin affinity which strengthens the interaction with the ECM.[5,6] In addition to talin, the kindlin family, a widely distributed PTB domain protein, has been recently involved in integrin activation (Fig. 1). In particular Kindlin-2 synergises with talin in integrin activation, behaving as an essential co-activator of integrin signaling.[7,8] In contrast to kindlin-2, kindlin-3 binds directly to regions of β-integrin tails distinct from those of talin, thus behaving as a novel element for platelet integrin activation in hemostasis and thrombosis.[9]

Two of the best-characterized focal adhesion proteins are vinculin and α-actinin. Vinculin is a ubiquitously expressed actin-binding protein characterized by a globular head and a tail domain

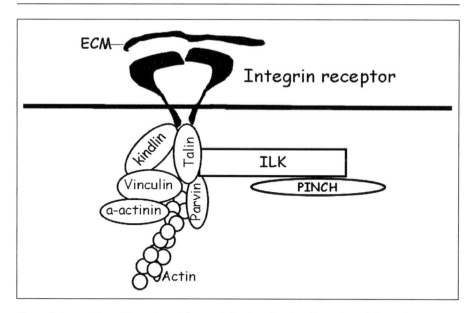

Figure 1. Interaction of integrins with cytoskeletal molecules. Overview of the major proteins by which integrins can link to the actin cytoskeleton. Talin and kindlin bind and activate integrins, while α-actinin, vinculin and the ILK/Pinch/Parvin complex recruits actin filaments to integrin clusters.

which interact each other to close the molecule in an inactive conformation masking the relevant ligand-binding sites. A-actinin is a cell-adhesion and cytoskeletal protein that cross-links actin filaments to bundles and networks linking these filaments directly to the integrin β subunit cytoplasmic domain. The cytoskeletal proteins belonging to the focal adhesion also interact one each other: for example α actinin binds vinculin as well as other proteins such as zyxin, Erk1/2, MEKK1 and the p85 subunit of phosphoinositide 3-kinase (PI-3K),[10] creating a relevant network of structural proteins.

An additional set of proteins involved in focal adhesion organisation is the IPP (ILK, Pinch, Parvin) complex.[11] Briefly, the ILK kinase is the central component of the IPP complex; it binds PINCH proteins through the N-terminal ankyrin-repeat domain and parvins through the kinase domain. It also links the complex to the cytoplasmic tails of β1 and β3 integrins. On the other side, parvin associates to vinculin and α-actinin. Although the complexity of this platform is beyond the scope of this chapter, the assembly of the IPP-complex precedes cell adhesion and is required for focal adhesion and cell spreading.

Regulation of most of the interactions originated in the focal adhesions are mediated through phosphoinositides binding. Phosphoinositides such as PIP2 have been shown to increase binding of talin to β1 integrin, by inducing a conformational change that un-masks the tail-binding site within the talin FERM domain. Upon integrin clustering, talin is recruited to focal complexes leading to the binding and activation of the PIP2-producing enzyme, the phosphatidylinositol phosphate kinase Type 1 gamma. Therefore talin can stimulate PIP2 local production, which leads to the association of talin.[12] Also for vinculin, the head-tail interaction that is characteristic of the inactive conformation, is removed by phosphoinositides, whose transient changes in the local concentrations stabilize vinculin in focal adhesions and thereby suppresses cell migration.[13] PIP2 binding also increases the interaction of vinculin and α actinin with actin, PKN and PI-3K, while PIP3 decreases the binding of α-actinin with integrins and regulates the interaction between parvin and ILK.

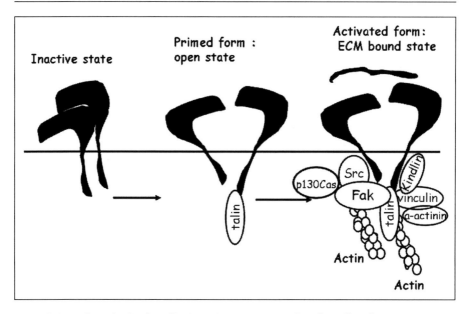

Figure 2. Integrin activation by talin. Integrins are expressed on the cell surface in an inactive and bend state. Upon talin binding the heterodimer undergoes conformational changes which induce cytoplasmic protein binding and reorganisation of the extracellular ligand binding pocket that increase affinity for ligands.

Integrin Signaling

Integrins are enzymatically inactive receptors, which link with cellular components to elicit signal transduction. Integrin ability to transduce signals inside the cells upon ECM binding, the so called "outside-in signaling" is required for polymerization of actin cytoskeleton during cell adhesion and for control of cell migration, proliferation, survival and differentiation. Direct evidence for a matrix-mediated intracellular signaling was provided in the late eighties by experiments showing that transcription of early response genes in quiescent fibroblasts or of genes related to the inflammatory response in monocytes are induced upon ECM interaction.[14,15]

Over the last twenty years more than 6000 papers have described the facets of "outside-in signaling". At the moment there is an expanded list of integrin-mediated signaling events which comprise most of the known signaling pathways. These include induction of cytosolic kinases, stimulation of the phosphainositides metabolism, activation of Ras/MAPK and PKC pathways and regulation of Rho GTPases.[16-19] These signals greatly overlap with those activated by growth factor and cytokine receptors. However, the extent and duration of each signals vary depending on whether the integrin, the growth factor receptors or both are engaged by the ligand, indicating that signals from integrin, growth factor and cytokine receptors are properly integrated. This view reflects the fact that in vivo, cells must integrate multiple stimuli from adhesions, growth factors, hormones and mechanical stresses to determine the appropriate response.

The SFK-Fak-p130Cas Signaling

As mentioned before, upon binding to the matrix, integrins undergo a conformational change and interact with signaling proteins to convey information to the nucleus. Tyrosine phosphorylation of proteins represents a primary response to integrin stimulation and a preferential way to transduce signals throughout the cell. Among the kinases that are activated and the proteins that are tyrosine phosphorylated upon ECM binding, the Src Family Kinases (SFKs), Focal adhesion kinase (Fak) and the adaptor molecule p130Cas play a prominent role in integrin signaling.

The Focal Adhesion Kinase

Fak is an evolutionary conserved 116 kDa scaffold protein that recruit cytoskeletal and signaling molecules involved in integrin-dependent events including cell migration, growth factor signaling, cell cycle progression and cell survival.[20-22] Fak contains distinct domains able to interact with several molecules, some of which drive its localization to focal adhesions, while others are implicated in downstream signaling. In addition to the central catalytic domain, the amino-terminal domain contains the tyrosine residue Tyr397, which is the primary site of auto catalytic phosphorylation and a FERM domain which interacts with the cytoplasmic tails of the β1 integrin and with activated growth factor receptors.[23] The carboxy-terminal region is characterized by two proline-rich domains that bind to SH3 containing proteins, such as p130Cas and the Tyr925 that binds to SH2 domains when phosphorylated. This domain also contains the Focal Adhesion Targeting (FAT) sequence, that is required for the localization of Fak to newly formed and existing adhesion complexes.[21] Upon integrin engagement trans-auto phosphorylation on Fak Tyr397 creates a site of high affinity interaction for the SH2 domain of the SFKs, the p85 regulatory subunit of PI-3K and the phospholipase C gamma. In addition phosphorylation of Tyr925 promotes its association with the SH2 domain of the Grb2 adaptor promoting signaling to MAPK.[21]

What is driving the choice between the different interacting molecules, or the contribution of each of them in the downstream signaling, is still an open question. It is likely that the timing of Fak activation and the recruitment of distinct downstream effectors vary in different cell compartments. Interestingly Fak has been recently reported to localize into the nucleus, where its FERM domain enhances Mdm2-dependent p53 ubiquitination, leading to FAK-dependent inactivation of p53.[24] The latter results support a novel biological role for nuclear Fak in promoting cell proliferation and survival by facilitating p53 turnover.

Src Family Kinases

The members of the Src family (Blk, Fgr, Fyn, Hck, Lck, Lyn, Src, Yes and Yrk) contain a regulatory Tyr527 in the carboxy-terminal tail, a SH1 kinase domain with the auto phosphorylation site on Tyr416, one SH2 and one SH3 domains regulating protein-protein interaction and a SH4 domain containing a myristylation site important for membrane localization.[25] In the inactive conformation, the molecule is closed by binding of the phosphorylated Tyr527 to the SH2 domain. Upon Tyr527 de-phosphorylation, the molecule opens up and is free for auto-phosphorylation and for interactions with downstream effectors. The balance between the inactive and the active form depends on activation of the Csk kinase which specifically phosphorylates the Tyr527, or de-phosphorylation events performed by PTPases such as PTPα and SHP1/2, but it might also occur in response to high levels of Src expression.[26] Recently the p140Cap adaptor protein has been demonstrated to act as a novel and potent regulator of Src kinase activity. Upon ECM binding, p140Cap activates Csk, which phosphorylates Src on Tyr527, resulting in inhibition of Src kinase activity and down-regulation of downstream signaling.[27]

Activated Src is translocated at the cell periphery at sites of cell adhesion, where it becomes associated to plasma membrane through its myristoylated domain, close to transmembrane tyrosine kinase receptors and integrins. In epithelial cells, active Src transiently associates with integrins in the early phases of cell adhesion.[28] In contrast in platelets Src has been shown to bind constitutively and selectively through its SH3 domain to the β3 integrin cytoplasmic tail.[29]

The p130Cas Adaptor Protein

p130Cas (Crk-associated substrate) is a scaffold protein originally identified as the major substrate of v-Src and v-Crk (30). p130Cas is characterized by a SH3 domain and a large substrate-binding domain containing 15 repeats of a YXXP sequence (tyrosine-any two aminoacids-proline), which serve as a tyrosine kinase substrate and, once phosphorylated, represent the binding site for SH2 or PTB domains of effectors proteins. The C-terminal domain contains a bipartite binding site that includes a proline-rich region that associates to the Src SH3 domain and a tyrosine containing sequence that could bind to the Src SH2 domain. Due to its ability to associate with multiple signaling partners, p130Cas is an important transducer of migratory and survival signals.

SFK-Fak-p130Cas as a Signaling Scaffold in Migration, Invasion and Survival

Upon integrin-mediated adhesion Fak, Src and p130Cas are associated in a multimeric signaling scaffold involved in the organization of focal adhesions and actin cytoskeleton and generation of signaling, ultimately regulating complex processes such as survival, motility, invasion and proliferation.

Upon migration, lamellipodia and filopodia are extended from the cell leading edge in the direction of migration creating new dynamic adhesions, which form and rapidly disassemble at the base of protrusions.[20,31] The use of live-cell imaging and expression of fluorescently labelled focal adhesion components to measure the rate constants for focal adhesion disassembly in live cells,[32] indicates that Fak, Src and p130Cas are all required for efficient disassembly of focal adhesions. Indeed tyrosine phosphorylation is required for focal adhesion turn-over and aberrant activation of Src kinases can profoundly affect the organization of focal adhesions leading to loss of cell spreading. Transformation by oncogenic v-Src correlates with disassembly of focal adhesions and with hyper-phosphorylation of integrins, p130Cas and Fak. By many approaches it has been shown that Src phosphorylates at least 10 out the 15 YXXP p130Cas sites.[33,34] Among these, tyrosine 331 is also phosphorylated by EGF receptor,[35] suggesting a direct effect of growth factors on p130Cas mediated cell migration. The current hypothesis is that upon Src activation and phosphorylation the assembly of a p130Cas/Crk/DOCK180 scaffold at adhesion sites drives localized Rac activation leading to actin polymerization and recruitment of high-affinity integrin receptors necessary for lamellipodia extension and cell migration.[36] To generate invasion, the Fak-Src-p130Cas-Dock180 signaling complex localised in lamellipodia activates also the JNK MAPK which induces matrix metalloproteinase expression and activity.

An additional mechanism by which Src and Fak can control focal adhesion organization and cell motility is the regulation of the small GTPase Rho. Integrin engagement leads to a transient decrease in RhoA activity, by a Src-dependent phosphorylation of p190RhoGAP causing a transient inactivation of RhoA. The latter relieves the contractile forces at the sites of integrin engagement leading to focal adhesion disruption and promoting lamellipodial extension during cell migration.[37] In conclusion, the following model can be proposed in which Src localizes at focal adhesions and by an SH2-mediated interaction with Fak, induces tyrosine phosphorylation of target molecules such as Fak itself and p130Cas, thus promoting actin skeleton organization, focal adhesion dynamic, cell motility and cell invasion.

Pro-survival signals emanating from the extracellular matrix (ECM) and soluble growth factors and hormones proceed via their respective receptors through FAK and Src to p130Cas to activate the small GTPases Ras and Rac as well as JNK and Erk1/2 MAPK.[30] p130Cas may also play a direct role in death signaling. Multiple pro-apoptotic stimuli, such as detachment from ECM (anoikis), treatment with anticancer drugs or UV irradiation, induce p130Cas cleavage by caspase-3 or other proteases, generating a C-terminal 31 kDa fragment. This fragment promotes loss of focal adhesions, cell rounding, nuclear condensation and fragmentation. It also contains an Helix-loop-helix domain that hetero-dimerizes with the transcription factor E2A and translocates to the cell nucleus, where it contributes to cell death by physically preventing E-box binding by E2A. Moreover the heterodimer inhibits E2A-mediated p21 transcription, thus promoting cell death.[30]

Integrin Cross Talk with Growth Factor and Cytokine Receptors

In addition to the pathways described above, growth factor and cytokine receptors and in particular receptor tyrosine kinase (RPTKs), are integrin partners in assembling the transduction machinery required for proliferation, survival and migration. Regulation of cell cycle is a prototypic event occurring by joint integrin/RPTKs signaling.[38] Normal cells need to adhere to the matrix to progress through the mid-G1 phase of the cell cycle upon mitogen treatment.[39] In adherent cells, the cascade of downstream events induced by soluble growth factors, such as EGF or PDGF, co-operates with that induced by integrins. Joint integrin/RPTKs signaling allows expression of cyclin D, activation of cyclin D-dependent kinases and degradation of Cdk inhibitor p27.[40] Integrins regulate RPTKs functions including receptor transactivation, co-ordination and compartmentalization and downstream signaling. Reciprocal cross-talk between integrins and the RPTKs consists in at least three hierarchical mechanisms, the first consisting in integrin ability to trigger ligand-independent RPTKs activation. On the other hand, integrins are also required for propagation of ligand-mediated signaling, leading to a full repertoire of RPTKs activities. In this case integrin and growth factor receptor signaling can act on parallel pathways and synergize to reach a final biological response. As a third possibility, integrins and their immediate target effectors can function as downstream transducers of RPTK signals.[18,41]

Integrins stimulates direct phosphorylation and partial activation of several RPTKs[16] in the absence of any growth factor ligand. The number of RPTKs involved suggests that this activation scheme can be a broadly used mechanism in adhesion-mediated signaling. In other words, cell-matrix adhesion represents a priming event and a limiting factor in addition to soluble ligand, for RPTKs activation.

In the case of the EGF receptor (EGFR), integrin-dependent activation leads to phosphorylation of EGFR on a specific subset of tyrosine residues, only partially overlapping with those phosphorylated by EGF. Upon adhesion, EGFR is phosphorylated on tyrosine 845, 1068, 1086 and 1173, but not on residue 1148, a major site of phosphorylation in response to EGF.[28,42,43] These data show that after integrin-dependent cell-ECM adhesion, the specific EGFR tyrosine residues that become phosphorylated do not correspond to all of the major sites previously shown to be phosphorylated by EGF, thus implying a differential activation of downstream signaling. Consistently, integrin-dependent EGFR activation induces cell survival as well as lamellipodia formation, cell spreading and migration, while is not sufficient for cell migration. In particular, integrin/EGFR signaling regulates the expression of the pro-apoptotic protein Bim, a critical mediator of anoikis in epithelial cells. In fact Bim is strongly induced after cell detachment by concomitant lack of β1 integrin engagement and down-regulation of EGFR expression.[44] Taken together, these data show that upon adhesion, EGFR trans-activation accounts for a specific repertoire of mechanisms, namely cell survival and actin cytoskeleton organization involved in cell migration.

The urokinase plasminogen activator receptor (uPAR), a GPI-linked protease receptor, has been shown to bind and activate α5β1 integrin and ERK signaling, inducing in vivo proliferation of HEp3 human carcinoma. Recent data show that this effect is mediated by adhesion-dependent EGFR trans-activation, unveiling a mechanism whereby uPAR by binding to integrins stimulates EGFR signaling, providing cancer cells with proliferative advantage.[45] In other cell systems, such as an in vivo hepatocyte tumour model, the ability of integrins to transactivate the HGF receptor Met is crucial for tumour metastasis, implying that cells could mistake signals form integrins, leading to inappropriate cell growth and tumourigenesis.[46]

Although much less investigated, similar mechanisms are depicted for integrin-dependent activation of cytokine receptors. The molecular mechanisms involved in such events include recruitment of crucial transducing proteins to membrane cytoskeletal complexes and enhancement of nuclear translocation of transcriptional regulators. Co-immunoprecipitation studies demonstrate that in endothelial cells the β common subunit of the IL-3 receptor (IL-3R) associates with the active β1 integrin. Upon adhesion to fibronectin JAK2 binds to this complex, is activated and leads to phosphorylation of the IL-3R and STAT5A,[47] giving further insights on the existence of an extensive integrin cross-talk including not only the tyrosine kinase but also the cytokine receptors.

Cooperation between Integrins, Growth Factor/Cytokine Receptors and Their Ligands: Reciprocal Potentiation

Integrins have been shown to potentiate signaling pathways in response to insulin, PDGF, EGF, FGF and VEGF (for reviews see 16,18). This co-operation begins at the level of the receptors themselves. In fact, cell adhesion increases the number of PDGF receptor by blocking their degradation by an ubiquitin-dependent pathway.[48] Many integrins form complexes with RPTKs and some appear to have preferred partners. For example, the αvβ3 integrin associates and synergizes with insulin, PDGF and VEGF receptors. B1 integrins associate with the EGFR and ErbB2; α6β4 combines with the EGFR, Erb-B2 and Met.[16] Interestingly, distinct integrin isoforms may selectively modulate RPTKs signaling. For example in response to IGF stimulation, the canonical β1A integrin associates with the insulin-like growth factor Type I receptor (IGF-IR) in a complex which support IGF-mediated cell proliferation. In contrast, β1C, an integrin cytoplasmic variant, completely prevents IGF-mediated cell proliferation and tumour growth by inhibiting IGF-IR auto-phosphorylation in response to IGF-I stimulation.[49] Therefore distinct integrin cytoplasmic domains finely tune growth factor signaling.

The co-operation between integrins and RPTKS is required to get full tyrosine phosphorylation of the receptors, their binding to signaling molecules and activation of downstream pathways (Fig. 3). In particular, combined activation of integrins and RPTKs is necessary to activate the Ras-ERK pathway beyond the threshold necessary for transcription of cyclin D.[50] This relies on the fact that integrin/RPTKs co-operation is required for enhancement of nuclear translocation of Erk1/2 transcriptional regulators and for efficient phosphorylation of the nuclear ERK substrate, Elk-1.[51] In terms of transcriptional response, β1 integrin is required for the early gene Egr-1 expression in response to EGF. This regulation occurs by integrin-dependent activation and nuclear translocation of Akt, which phosphorylates and inactivates the transcriptional regulator Forkhead, whose removal from the nucleus allows Egr-1 expression.[69]

The third mechanisms by which integrins and RPTKs undergo reciprocal regulation consists in the fact that integrins and their immediate target effectors can function as downstream transducers of RPTK signals to regulate cell migration. In particular, upon growth factor stimulation, Fak interacts with the RPTKs and with talin at integrin attachment sites,[23,52] bridging the two receptor systems. The relevance of Fak in RPTK-dependent regulation is highlighted by the observation that fibroblasts lacking Fak are refractory to PDGF and EGF-induced migration. In endothelial cells, Fak is constitutively associated with β1 and β3 integrins in the presence or absence of growth factors, but VEGF promotes the Src-mediated phosphorylation of Fak and its coupling to the αvβ5,[53] further supporting the concept that RPTKs can induce coupling of Fak to integrins.

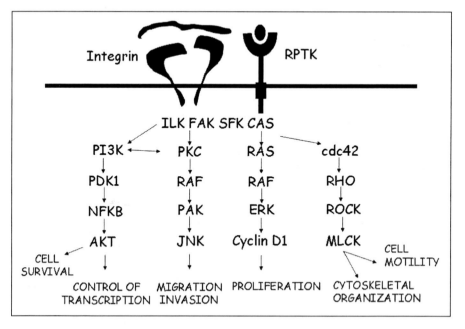

Figure 3. Signalling pathways emanating from integrins. Upon integrin binding to the ECM, the Fak/Src/p130Cas and the ILK complexes are assembled at the integrin sites, giving rise to many signalling pathways. The major signal transduction pathways and many of the key players in them are shown, leading to the effects on cell behaviour mediated by integrins, often acting in concert with RPTK receptors for soluble factors.

As a last example, in migrating epithelial and carcinoma cells the α6β4 integrin redistributes with motility structures and mediates cell movement. This peculiar integrin has been shown to associate with the EGFR and Met, that upon binding to their ligands, phosphorylate the β4 cytoplasmic domain and recruit Shc and PI-3K.[54,55] This event generates a signaling platform that potentiates EGF/HGF-triggered activation of Ras- and PI3K-dependent pathways, promoting cell motility and invasion. These observations highlight the fact that the β4 integrin can constitute a parallel docking platform that co-operates with RPTKs to amplify the signaling machinery.

Integrin Signaling and Cancer

The formation of integrin-dependent signaling complexes has increasing importance in tumour cell biology.[56] Both integrins and their major intracellular effectors such as ILK, Fak, p130Cas or Src have been shown to control tumourigenesis in various animal models of cancers. Most of the data have been collected in breast cancer models. Targeted ablation of β1 or Fak in the mammary gland provides a direct demonstration that these two molecules are required both in initiation and maintenance of in vivo mammary tumour growth induced by Polyoma virus.[57,58] Over-expression of the integrin effector ILK under the MMTV promoter in the mouse mammary gland results in the formation of spontaneous focal mammary tumours, while over-expression of p130Cas and Src in the same system induces mammary gland hyperplasia and acceleration of ErbB2-dependent tumourigenesis.[70] As a last example, loss of β4 signaling suppresses mammary tumour onset and invasive growth by amplifying ErbB2 signaling.[60,61]

In addition, mouse models have shown that integrins are required also for metastatic dissemination of primary tumours to secondary tissues. The specific role that integrins play during mammary tumour metastasis in experimental mouse models has been suggested from cell culture-based systems, both in 2D and 3D reconstituted matrices. The results of these experiments, combined with correlative studies on human breast cancer samples, suggest that integrins are involved at all stages of metastasis, including tumour cell migration, invasion and colonization of target tissues.[62,63] As with tumour cell growth and normal mammary gland physiology, the impact of integrin expression on breast cancer metastasis has again been shown to involve multimolecular adhesion complexes. The formation of these complexes confers to integrins the ability to mediate the biological response to diverse physiological signals important for invasion and metastasis.

Important insight into the role of integrins in metastasis has also been gained from the analysis of other tumour cell types, such as lung and pancreatic tumour cells. Lung metastasis from an experimental xenograft model of human breast cancer, for example, were shown to be impaired following systemic administration of an inhibitory anti-β1 integrin antibody.[64] Similarly, administration of a peptide designed to block the α5β1 and αvβ3 receptors was found to impair the growth and metastasis of invasive human breast cancer cells.[65] In the Rip1Tag2 transgenic mouse model of pancreatic β cell carcinogenesis ablation of β1 integrin in β cells resulted in impaired primary tumour growth by a defect in cell proliferation and dissemination of tumour cell emboli into lymphatic blood vessels. However disseminating β1 integrin-deficient β tumour cells did not elicit metastasis.[66]

It has been well established that a tumour in order to keep growing is dependent on a continuous blood supply and thus neoangiogenesis is one of the most important collateral processes that are stimulated by tumour cells. In this regard, alterations of expression of various integrins and downstream signaling molecules have been observed in various cancers, in particular those in which angiogenesis is known to play a prominent role.[67] Inhibition of specific integrins might thus reduce both the direct effects of integrins on cancer cells and in a more indirect way tumour angiogenesis.

In addition to a direct role of integrins in the onset and maintenance of tumourigenesis, integrin-mediated adhesion of cells to ECM proteins is also very relevant for inducing an increased cell survival after exposure to chemotherapy and ionizing radiation in vitro.[22] This mechanism might be in part causative for radiation and chemoresistance phenotypes in tumour cells. B1 integrins have been implicated in mediating resistance to cytotoxic chemotherapy and radiation. Elevated integrin cell surface expression has been detected in irradiated tumour cells and correlated with an increase in cell adhesion and activation of MMPs. In the contest of a tissue, this might have specific consequences for invasion and metastasis influencing tumour growth and patient's survival.

As a consequence, inhibitory peptides, anti-integrin monoclonal antibodies and non peptide chemical integrin antagonists[68] are currently being investigated in clinical trials in patients with solid tumours. Evidences suggest clinical benefit in disease stabilization with use of an anti-αVbeta3 antibody in the settings of glioblastoma, melanoma, colorectal, renal, breast, prostate and lung cancer. Integrin inhibition by antagonists interferes with binding to ECM thereby preventing survival and proliferation signals. Therefore targeted treatment with these antagonists might be highly effective as an adjuvant therapy in combination with other therapeutic approaches in solid cancer patients.

Conclusion

The picture emerging from these studies is that integrins behave as nodes within webs of signaling, adhesive and cytoskeletal pathways. In conclusion, integrins exert most prominent signaling functions through the activation of cytoplasmic kinases such as SFKs and Fak, cross-talk with growth factor and cytokine receptors and building up of transducing macromolecular complexes with adaptor molecules. Each of the partners brings a distinctive contribution to downstream signaling and it will be important to elucidate in the next future the mechanisms by which they associate and those by which they respond to extracellular signals to induce and integrate a cellular response. These mechanisms can also be translated in a clinical set in many pathologies where integrin signaling has been altered.

Acknowledgement

This work was supported by grants of the Italian Association for Cancer Research (AIRC), Association for International Cancer Research (AICR), EU FP7 program Metafight, MUR (Ministero dell'Università e Ricerca Scientifica, cofinanziamento PRIN, fondi ex-60%), Special project "Oncology", Compagnia San Paolo/FIRM, Torino, Italy, Regione Piemonte-Progetti Sanitá, Oncoprot and Progetto Alfieri, Fondazione CRT, Torino, Italy.

References

1. Hynes RO. The emergence of integrins: a personal and historical perspective. Matrix Biol 2004; 23:333-40.
2. Sastry SK, Burridge K. Focal adhesions: a nexus for intracellular signaling and cytoskeletal dynamics. Exp Cell Res 2000; 261:25-36.
3. Lock JG, Wehrle-Haller B, Stromblad S. Cell-matrix adhesion complexes: master control machinery of cell migration. Semin Cancer Biol 2008; 18:65-76.
4. Arnaout MA, Goodman SL, Xiong JP. Structure and mechanics of integrin-based cell adhesion. Curr Opin Cell Biol 2007; 19:495-507.
5. Garcia-Alvarez B, de Pereda JM, Calderwood DA et al. Structural determinants of integrin recognition by talin. Mol Cell 2003; 11:49-58.
6. Vinogradova O, Velyvis A, Velyviene A et al. A structural mechanism of integrin α(IIb)beta(3) "inside-out" activation as regulated by its cytoplasmic face. Cell 2002; 110:587-97.
7. Ma YQ, Qin J, Wu C et al. Kindlin-2 (Mig-2): a co-activator of beta3 integrins. J Cell Biol 2008; 181:439-46.
8. Montanez E, Ussar S, Schifferer M et al. Kindlin-2 controls bidirectional signaling of integrins. Genes Dev 2008; 22:1325-30.
9. Moser M, Nieswandt B, Ussar S et al. Kindlin-3 is essential for integrin activation and platelet aggregation. Nat Med 2008; 14:325-30.
10. Brakebusch C, Fassler R. The integrin-actin connection, an eternal love affair. EMBO J 2003; 22:2324-33.
11. Legate KR, Montanez E, Kudlacek O et al. ILK, PINCH and parvin: the tIPP of integrin signaling. Nat Rev Mol Cell Biol 2006; 7:20-31.
12. Nayal A, Webb DJ, Horwitz AF. Talin: an emerging focal point of adhesion dynamics. Curr Opin Cell Biol 2004; 16:94-8.
13. Ziegler WH, Liddington RC, Critchley DR. The structure and regulation of vinculin. Trends Cell Biol 2006; 16:453-60.
14. Dike LE, Farmer SR. Cell adhesion induces expression of growth-associated genes in suspension-arrested fibroblasts. Proc Natl Acad Sci USA 1988; 85:6792-6.

15. Eierman DF, Johnson CE, Haskill JS. Human monocyte inflammatory mediator gene expression is selectively regulated by adherence substrates. J Immunol 1989; 142:1970-6.
16. Defilippi P, Tarone G, Gismondi A, Santoni A, eds. Integrins and Signal Transduction. Austin/New York: Landes Bioscience/Springer, 2006.
17. Giancotti FG, Tarone G. Positional control of cell fate through joint integrin/receptor protein kinase signaling. Annu Rev Cell Dev Biol 2003; 19:173-206.
18. Miranti CK, Brugge JS. Sensing the environment: a historical perspective on integrin signal transduction. Nat Cell Biol 2002; 4:E83-90.
19. Schwartz MA, Ginsberg MH. Networks and crosstalk: integrin signalling spreads. Nat Cell Biol 2002; 4:E65-8.
20. Mitra SK, Schlaepfer DD. Integrin-regulated FAK-Src signaling in normal and cancer cells. Curr Opin Cell Biol 2006; 18:516-23.
21. Parsons JT. Focal adhesion kinase: the first ten years. J Cell Sci 2003; 116:1409-16.
22. van Nimwegen MJ, van de Water B. Focal adhesion kinase: a potential target in cancer therapy. Biochem Pharmacol 2007; 73:597-609.
23. Sieg DJ, Hauck CR, Ilic D et al. FAK integrates growth-factor and integrin signals to promote cell migration. Nat Cell Biol 2000; 2:249-56.
24. Lim ST, Chen XL, Lim Y et al. Nuclear FAK promotes cell proliferation and survival through FERM-enhanced p53 degradation. Mol Cell 2008; 29:9-22.
25. Yeatman TJ. A renaissance for SRC. Nat Rev Cancer 2004; 4:470-80.
26. Irby RB, Mao W, Coppola D et al. Activating SRC mutation in a subset of advanced human colon cancers. Nat Genet 1999; 21:187-90.
27. Di Stefano P, Damiano L, Cabodi S et al. p140Cap protein suppresses tumour cell properties, regulating Csk and Src kinase activity. EMBO J 2007; 26:2843-55.
28. Moro L, Dolce L, Cabodi S et al. Integrin-induced epidermal growth factor (EGF) receptor activation requires c-Src and p130Cas and leads to phosphorylation of specific EGF receptor tyrosines. J Biol Chem 2002; 277:9405-14.
29. de Virgilio M, Kiosses WB, Shattil SJ. Proximal, selective and dynamic interactions between integrin alphaIIbbeta3 and protein tyrosine kinases in living cells. J Cell Biol 2004; 165:305-11.
30. Defilippi P, Di Stefano P, Cabodi S. p130Cas: a versatile scaffold in signaling networks. Trends Cell Biol 2006; 16:257-63.
31. Ridley AJ, Schwartz MA, Burridge K et al. Cell migration: integrating signals from front to back. Science 2003; 302:1704-9.
32. Webb DJ, Donais K, Whitmore LA et al. FAK-Src signalling through paxillin, ERK and MLCK regulates adhesion disassembly. Nat Cell Biol 2004; 6:154-61.
33. Goldberg GS, Alexander DB, Pellicena P et al. Src phosphorylates Cas on tyrosine 253 to promote migration of transformed cells. J Biol Chem 2003; 278:46533-40.
34. Shin NY, Dise RS, Schneider-Mergener J et al. Subsets of the major tyrosine phosphorylation sites in Crk-associated substrate (CAS) are sufficient to promote cell migration. J Biol Chem 2004; 279:38331-7.
35. Zhang XT, Li LY, Mu XL et al. The EGFR mutation and its correlation with response of gefitinib in previously treated Chinese patients with advanced nonsmall-cell lung cancer. Ann Oncol 2005; 16:1334-42.
36. Burridge K, Wennerberg K. Rho and Rac take center stage. Cell 2004; 116:167-79.
37. Chang LC, Huang CH, Cheng CH et al. Differential effect of the focal adhesion kinase Y397F mutant on v-Src-stimulated cell invasion and tumor growth. J Biomed Sci 2005; 12:571-85.
38. Schwartz MA, Assoian RK. Integrins and cell proliferation: regulation of cyclin-dependent kinases via cytoplasmic signaling pathways. J Cell Sci 2001; 114:2553-60.
39. Assoian RK. Control of the G1 phase cyclin-dependent kinases by mitogenic growth factors and the extracellular matrix. Cytokine Growth Factor Rev 1997; 8:165-70.
40. Carrano AC, Pagano M. Role of the F-box protein Skp2 in adhesion-dependent cell cycle progression. J Cell Biol 2001; 153:1381-90.
41. Comoglio PM, Boccaccio C, Trusolino L. Interactions between growth factor receptors and adhesion molecules: breaking the rules. Curr Opin Cell Biol 2003; 15:565-71.
42. Boeri Erba E, Bergatto E, Cabodi S et al. Systematic analysis of the epidermal growth factor receptor by mass spectrometry reveals stimulation-dependent multisite phosphorylation. Mol Cell Proteomics 2005; 4:1107-21.
43. Boeri Erba E, Matthiesen R, Bunkenborg J et al. Quantitation of multisite EGF receptor phosphorylation using mass spectrometry and a novel normalization approach. J Proteome Res 2007; 6:2768-85.
44. Reginato MJ, Mills KR, Paulus JK et al. Integrins and EGFR coordinately regulate the pro-apoptotic protein Bim to prevent anoikis. Nat Cell Biol 2003; 5:733-40.

45. Monaghan-Benson E, McKeown-Longo PJ. Urokinase-type plasminogen activator receptor regulates a novel pathway of fibronectin matrix assembly requiring Src-dependent transactivation of epidermal growth factor receptor. J Biol Chem 2006; 281:9450-9.
46. Wang R, Ferrell LD, Faouzi S et al. Activation of the Met receptor by cell attachment induces and sustains hepatocellular carcinomas in transgenic mice. J Cell Biol 2001; 153:1023-34.
47. Defilippi P, Rosso A, Dentelli P et al. {beta}1 Integrin and IL-3R coordinately regulate STAT5 activation and anchorage-dependent proliferation. J Cell Biol 2005; 168:1099-108.
48. Baron V, Schwartz M. Cell adhesion regulates ubiquitin-mediated degradation of the platelet-derived growth factor receptor beta. J Biol Chem 2000; 275:39318-23.
49. Goel HL, Fornaro M, Moro L et al. Selective modulation of type 1 insulin-like growth factor receptor signaling and functions by beta1 integrins. J Cell Biol 2004; 166:407-18.
50. Roovers K, Assoian RK. Integrating the MAP kinase signal into the G1 phase cell cycle machinery. Bioessays 2000; 22:818-26.
51. Aplin AE, Stewart SA, Assoian RK et al. Integrin-mediated adhesion regulates ERK nuclear translocation and phosphorylation of Elk-1. J Cell Biol 2001; 153:273-82.
52. Ivankovic-Dikic I, Gronroos E, Blaukat A et al. Pyk2 and FAK regulate neurite outgrowth induced by growth factors and integrins. Nat Cell Biol 2000; 2:574-81.
53. Eliceiri BP, Puente XS, Hood JD et al. Src-mediated coupling of focal adhesion kinase to integrin alpha(v) beta5 in vascular endothelial growth factor signaling. J Cell Biol 2002; 157:149-60.
54. Mariotti A, Kedeshian PA, Dans M et al. EGF-R signaling through Fyn kinase disrupts the function of integrin alpha6beta4 at hemidesmosomes: role in epithelial cell migration and carcinoma invasion. J Cell Biol 2001; 155:447-58.
55. Trusolino L, Bertotti A, Comoglio PM. A signaling adapter function for alpha6beta4 integrin in the control of HGF-dependent invasive growth. Cell 2001; 107:643-54.
56. Hehlgans S, Haase M, Cordes N. Signalling via integrins: implications for cell survival and anticancer strategies. Biochim Biophys Acta 2007; 1775:163-80.
57. Lahlou H, Sanguin-Gendreau V, Zuo D et al. Mammary epithelial-specific disruption of the focal adhesion kinase blocks mammary tumor progression. Proc Natl Acad Sci USA 2007; 104:20302-7.
58. White DE, Kurpios NA, Zuo D et al. Targeted disruption of beta1-integrin in a transgenic mouse model of human breast cancer reveals an essential role in mammary tumor induction. Cancer Cell 2004; 6:159-70.
59. Guy CT, Muthuswamy SK, Cardiff RD et al. Activation of the c-Src tyrosine kinase is required for the induction of mammary tumors in transgenic mice. Genes Dev 1994; 8:23-32.
60. Guo W, Pylayeva Y, Pepe A et al. Beta 4 integrin amplifies ErbB2 signaling to promote mammary tumorigenesis. Cell 2006; 126:489-502.
61. Bon G, Folgiero V, Di Carlo S et al. Involvement of alpha6beta4 integrin in the mechanisms that regulate breast cancer progression. Breast Cancer Res 2007; 9:203.
62. Brakebusch C, Fassler R. beta 1 integrin function in vivo: adhesion, migration and more. Cancer Metastasis Rev 2005; 24:403-11.
63. Christofori G. New signals from the invasive front. Nature 2006; 441:444-50.
64. Elliott BE, Ekblom P, Pross H et al. Anti-beta 1 integrin IgG inhibits pulmonary macrometastasis and the size of micrometastases from a murine mammary carcinoma. Cell Adhes Commun 1994; 1:319-32.
65. Khalili P, Arakelian A, Chen G et al. A nonRGD-based integrin binding peptide (ATN-161) blocks breast cancer growth and metastasis in vivo. Mol Cancer Ther 2006; 5:2271-80.
66. Kren A, Baeriswyl V, Lehembre F et al. Increased tumor cell dissemination and cellular senescence in the absence of beta1-integrin function. EMBO J 2007; 26:2832-42.
67. Serini G, Napione L, Arese M et al. Besides adhesion: new perspectives of integrin functions in angiogenesis. Cardiovasc Res 2008; 78:213-22.
68. Huveneers S, Truong H, Danen HJ. Integrins: signaling, disease and therapy. Int J Radiat Biol 2007; 83:743-51.
69. Cabodi S, Morello V, Masi A et al. Convergence of integrins and EGF receptor signaling via PI3K/Akt/ FoxO pathway in early gene Egr-1 expression. J Cell Physiol. 2009; 218:294-303.
70. Cabodi S, Tinnirello A, Di Stefano P et al. p130Cas as a new regulator of mammary epithelial cell proliferation, survival, and HER2-neu oncogene-dependent breast tumorigenesis. Cancer Res. 2006; 1:4672-4680.

CHAPTER 6

Physical and Functional Interaction between Integrins and hERG1 Channels in Cancer Cells

Serena Pillozzi and Annarosa Arcangeli*

Abstract

Cancer is a complex multistep disease characterized by a profound genetic instability which leads to the aberrant and uncoordinated expression of several gene products, ultimately leading to the acquisition of a malignant phenotype. The identification of molecules and pathways that contribute to cancer establishment and progression has determined an enormous progress in oncology, providing new perspectives for the design of more specific and efficacious pharmacological approaches.

In this picture, ion channels represent a relatively novel and unexpected player. In fact, the expression and activity of different channel types mark and regulate specific stages of cancer progression. The contribution of ion channels to the neoplastic phenotype ranges from the control of cell proliferation and apoptosis, to the regulation of invasiveness and metastatic spread. The role of ion channels in such processes can often be attributed to novel signaling mechanisms triggered and modulated by ion channel proteins, independently from ion fluxes.

Ion channels encoded by the *human ether-à-go-go-related gene 1* (*herg1*), hERG1 channels, are often aberrantly expressed in many primary human cancers and exert pleiotropic effects in cancer cells. Some of them are strictly related to the modulation of adhesive interactions with the extracellular matrix. The latter in turn can either regulate cell differentiation, or improve cell motility and invasiveness or stimulate the process of neo-angiogenesis. hERG1 channels can induce such diverse effects since they trigger and modulate intracellular signaling cascades. This role often depends on the formation, on the plasma membrane of tumor cells, of macromolecular complexes with membrane receptors, especially integrins. The link between hERG1 and integrins is twofold: integrins, mainly the β1 integrin subunit, can activate hERG1. Conversely, the channels, once activated by integrins, can modulate signaling pathways downstream to integrin receptors.

Both effects are mediated by the formation of a hERG1/β1 integrin complex. Based on current evidence, we hypothesize that the activity of hERG1 channels inside the complex modulates the function of the partner protein(s) mainly through conformational coupling, instead of alterations of ion flow. Moreover, the hERG1-centered plasma membrane complexes, being specific of cancer cells, could represent novel targets for antineoplastic therapy.

*Corresponding Author: Annarosa Arcangeli—Department of Experimental Pathology and Oncology, University of Firenze. Viale G.B. Morgagni, 50, 50134 Firenze, Italy. Email: annarosa.arcangeli@unifi.it

Integrins and Ion Channels: Molecular Complexes and Signaling, edited by Andrea Becchetti and Annarosa Arcangeli. ©2010 Landes Bioscience and Springer Science+Business Media.

Introduction

Cancer is a multistep process, characterized by the progressive accumulation of genetic defects (somatic mutations, over expression of cancer related genes, inactivation or deletion of tumor suppressor genes) that ultimately leads to the acquisition of an uncontrolled malignancy.[1] In the last two decades, increasing evidences have indicated that different types of ion channels are involved in tumor establishment and progression (reviewed in references 2,3). Ion channels can contribute to the neoplastic phenotype at different steps of tumor progression. Most results point to the implication of K$^+$ channels in the control of cell proliferation and survival.[4-6] Additionally, a variety of Na$^+$, K$^+$ and Cl$^-$ channels, also profoundly affect cancer cell motility and invasion.[7-12] Their expression confers a more malignant phenotype, thus marking later, invasive and metastatic, stages of tumor progression. Importantly, evidence has been provided indicating that both tumor cell proliferation and invasion can be halted by the use of channel blockers (reviewed in 2). In this light, ion channel blockers have been recently tested in vivo in both preclinical models and in the clinical setting, with promising results.[2,13,14]

The mechanisms by which ion channels exert such pleiotropic functions in cancer are manifold. One possibility is that the K$^+$ channels control of the resting Vm regulates Ca^{2+} influx and thus the [Ca^{2+}]-dependent cell cycle checkpoints. This has been proven only in certain blood cells, but could be of general occurrence.[6] In addition, specific nonconductive roles of individual ion channel types on both tumor cell proliferation and invasion cannot be excluded.[2] These nonconductive ion-channel roles could be more or less dependent on the classic effects on V$_m$, depending on whether the intracellular modulatory domains of the channel protein are conformationally associated or not with the gating process. In different contexts, coordination or disengagement of the electric and biochemical roles could occur. For example, channels belonging to the *ether-à-go-go* (EAG) family of outward rectifying K$^+$ channels, the EAG-1 channels, stimulate proliferation in vitro, in a way that depends on channel conformational state, but not on ion conduction.[15] A complex and interesting signaling network is thus emerging, with ion channels effects on V$_m$ possibly modulating the cell machinery not so much (or not always) because of changes in ion fluxes, but through the mediation of voltage-dependent conformational changes that affect other cellular proteins, including membrane receptors of different kinds. Although the relation of these mechanisms with the cellular physiopathology is only beginning to be unravelled, such a bifunctional nature of ion channels could help to explain the great variety of channel expression profiles observed in cancer. Aggressive tumor cell clones may select certain ion channels because of their specific nonconductive signaling roles, both during early and late stages of the neoplastic progression. Such roles can somehow be ascribed to the physical and functional link between ion channels and adhesion receptors, mainly those belonging to the integrin family.[16]

In the present chapter we will describe hERG1, one of the K$^+$ channels most commonly expressed in cancer cells, focusing on the relevance of its interaction with integrin receptors for neoplasia.

hERG1 Channels in Cancer Cells

We and other groups have provided evidence that both human tumor cell lines and primary human cancers of different histogenesis express functional hERG1 channels.[17] hERG1 is encoded by the *herg1* gene, which belongs to an evolutionarily conserved multigenic family of voltage-activated, outward rectifying K$^+$ channels, the *EAG* family.[18] It is normally expressed in the heart,[19] as well as in selected neuronal and endocrine populations,[20] whereas it is absent in the majority of normal epithelial and mesenchymal cells, at least in the adult.[21,22]

The molecular structure of hERG1 channels is typical of the so called "six transmembrane domain" (6TM) ion channels. As is the case for the other voltage-gated K$^+$ channels, hERG1 is a tetramer of polypeptide subunits, each spanning six times the plasma membrane and containing a "P loop" between the fifth and sixth transmembrane domains, that lines the extracellular side of the channel pore. Both the N- and C- termini of the protein are located intracellularly. The N-terminus contains a Per-Arnt-Sym (PAS) domain at the very beginning of the polypeptide chain and a hERG1-specific proximal Domain (PD), close to the first transmembrane segment

(S1). Although it has not been proven yet for hERG1, the PAS domain is generally involved in protein-protein interactions that mediate sensing of environmental signals in prokaryotes and transcriptional regulation in eukaryotes. The C-terminus contains a cyclic nucleotide binding domain (cNBD), as well as specific amino acid sequences which are necessary for the recapitulation of the protein on the plasma membrane.[23] The above features define the "classical", full length product of the *herg1* gene, located on chromosome 7q35.36, whose mutations may cause the inherited form of the long QT syndrome.[24] Different splicing products and/or alternative transcripts have also been described. For example, we first described the *herg1b* alternative transcript in human leukemia and neuroblastoma cells.[25] *Herg1b* encodes for a protein, hERG1B, that shows a deleted N-terminus, where the PAS and PD domains are substituted by a short stretch of hydrophilic aminoacids. *Herg1b* is also expressed in the human heart.[26] In the heart *herg1* is expressed at higher levels compared to *herg1b*.[27] On the contrary, in tumor cells, the *herg1b* transcript often prevails[27,28] and hERG1B forms heterotetramers with hERG1,[25] thus dictating the biophysical features of the resulting current (Wanke E. et al, personal communication). The molecular structures of hERG1 and hERG1B are presented in Figure 1.

While *herg1b* is an alternative transcript, with its own promoter region, a splice product of the *herg1* gene was identified by Kuppershmidt et al[29] and named *herg1*$_{USO}$. The *herg1*$_{USO}$ transcript presents an unique exon at the 3' end, the USO exon, that substitutes most of the intracytoplasmic C-terminus, encoded by exons 9 to 15, with a small stretch of aminoacids. More recently we cloned and characterized a new *herg1* transcript, which contains the *1b* exon at the 5' end and the USO exon at the 3' end and hence was named *herg1b*$_{USO}$.[27] The proteins encoded from both transcripts, hERG1$_{USO}$ and hERG1B$_{USO}$, do not give rise to any detectable ion current, since they are not expressed on the plasma membrane, but are retained in the endoplasmic reticulum. Interestingly,

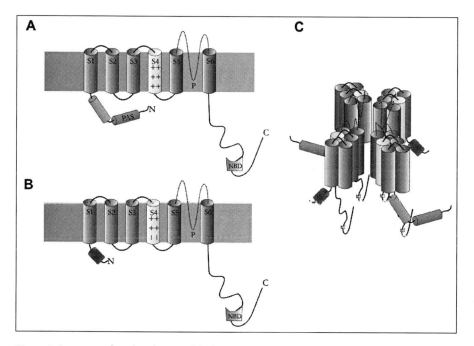

Figure 1. Structure of single subunits of the hERG1(A) and hERG1B (B) proteins. The two proteins can form homo- or hetero-tetramers onto the plasma membrane. The latter is shown in (C). Abbreviations: PAS: Per-Arnt-Sym domain; NBD: cyclic nucleotide binding domain; S1-S6: transmembrane domains; P: channel pore. The + in the S4 domain represent positively charged aminoacids in the voltage sensor.

hERG1B$_{USO}$ accomplishes a fundamental function in cancer cells, since it regulates hERG1 channel surface expression through a very peculiar posttranslational mechanism. In fact, hERG1B$_{USO}$ can form heterotetramers with either of the two full length hERG1 proteins (hERG1 and hERG1B). The heterotetramers are retained intracellularly and undergo ubiquitin-dependent degradation. This process results in decreased hERG1 current density in cancer cells. The hERG1B$_{USO}$-dependent control of hERG1 current density is apparently a check point in the regulation of different functions in cancers cells, from cell differentiation to apoptosis.[27]

In the heart, hERG1 currents contribute to the repolarization of the cardiac action potential[23] and in neurons regulate spike-frequency adaptation.[30-32] What is the role of hERG1 currents in cancer cells? Which biophysical characteristic of hERG1 makes it them so relevant in tumor cell behaviour? For our purposes, it is sufficient to note that because of the crossover of activation and inactivation curves, hERG1 produces steady state currents around −40 mV[33] and can determine tonic modulation of both excitable (firing threshold) and non-excitable (resting potential) cells. The range of V$_m$ between −30 and −50 mV is particularly relevant for cycling cells.[34] Moreover, when hERG1 currents are mainly sustained by hERG1B channels, they display a faster rate of activation and inactivation and hence steady state currents fit to sustain more depolarized values (−20 mV).[27,35] This is indeed the V$_m$ value of many tumor cells, especially leukemias.[35] In addition, at least in certain neuroblastoma cells, hERG1B is significantly up regulated during the S phase of the cell cycle and this could account for the depolarized V$_m$ value detected in cycling cells.[25]

Herg1 can be considered a proliferation related gene, at least in leukemia,[28,36,37] neuroblastoma[25] and gastric cancer cells.[38-40] In these cell types, the addition of drugs that specifically block the conductive activity of hERG1 channels (Class III antiarrhythmic drugs like E 4031 or Way 123,398, antibiotics like erythromycin, antihistaminics like torfenadine or the pro kinetic cisapride)[41,42] impairs cell proliferation. At least in leukemia cells, such impairment is due to the block of the cells in the G1 phase of the cell cycle.[36] The pro-proliferative role of hERG1 channels in leukemia cells was also supported by the demonstration that leukemia cell lines and primary leukemia blasts expressing different levels of hERG1 show a different capacity to engraft the bone marrow, when injected into immunodeficient mice.[28] This fact can be related to a hERG1-dependent autocrine regulation of VEGF-A secretion and hence of cell survival and proliferation. A similar hERG1-dependent regulation of VEGF-A secretion was shown also in glioblastoma[43] and gastric cancer cells (Lastraioli E., personal communication). However, in leukemia cells, the role of hERG1 channels is by far more complex, since their activity also affects cell migration outside the bone marrow and hence into the peripheral blood and extramedullary organs. On the whole, *herg1* expression in leukemia cells appears to represent a crucial step in the malignant phenotype progression.[28] A similar picture can also be applied to colorectal cancer, where the amount of functional hERG1 channels expressed on the plasma membrane is an important determinant for the acquisition of an invasive phenotype.[9] This correlates with the highest incidence of hERG1 expression in invasive and metastatic colorectal adenocarcinomas, with no expression in adenomas.[9] A different role is apparently exerted by hERG1 channels in neoplastic lesions of the upper gastrointestinal tract. In fact, hERG1 was found to be expressed in precancerous lesions of both the stomach and the lower tract of the esophagus and its expression predicts later progression towards a true cancer.[44]

In summary, a progressively more defined picture is emerging, in which hERG1 is expressed in several types of human cancers and exert different effects on tumor cell behaviour, often with a tissue specificity (see Table 1). Such specificity could depend on the binding to the *herg1* promoter of different cancer-specific transcription factors. Indeed, the *herg1* promoter does contain binding sites for several oncogenes and tumor suppressor genes.[45] What about the different effects of hERG1 channels in tumor cells? It is difficult to hypothesize that hERG1 channels could differently regulate V$_m$ dynamics in so many different tumor types. It is perhaps more likely that such a variety of effects could depend on cell-specific signaling pathways switched on or modulated by hERG1 channels, dependent or not from K$^+$ fluxes and V$_m$ alterations. We can thus consider hERG1 channels as bifunctional proteins,[2] in that they can both regulate V$_m$ and modulate different membrane or cytosolic proteins in both voltage-dependent and voltage-independent ways. One

Table 1. hERG1 expression in neoplastic cell lines and primary samples

Tumor	Mechamism of Expression in Tumors	Role in Tumor Progression	Mechanism of Action in Tumors	References
Leukemia	Over expression. Presence of splice variants and alternative transcripts	Control of cell differentiation. Control of cell proliferation and invasion. Contribution to chemoresistance. Correlation with shorter overall survival in primary myeloid leukemias	Formation of molecular complexes with β1 integrin and GF(growth factor) or chemokine receptors. Modulation of signaling pathways	28,36,48,58
Neuroblastoma	Presence of splice variants and alternative transcripts	Control of cell differentiation. Control of cell proliferation	Formation of molecular complexes with β1 integrin	25,33,46,47
Brain	Altered expression in glial tumors and glial tumor cells	Correlation to tumor grade	Modulation of VEGF-A secretion.	43
Colon	Over expression in primary colorectal cancers	Control of cell invasion and marker of advanced stages	Formation of molecular complex with β1 integrin.	9
Stomach	Over expression in primary gastric cancers. Expression in precancerous lesions	Control of cell cycle and VEGF-A secretion.	Transcriptional control of *vegf-a*.	39,44

of the partners that are physically and functionally linked to hERG1 channels are represented by adhesion receptors belonging to the integrin family[16](see below).

Effects of Integrin Activation on hERG1 Channels

In general, the functional association between ion channels and integrins can rely on two different mechanisms: an effect of integrins on ion channel function ("outside-to-in") and, vice versa, a modulatory effect of ion channel activity on integrin function and signaling ("inside-to-out"). In different experimental systems either of the two mechanisms can occur.[16] When hERG1 channels are involved in the cross talk with integrins, a complex interplay between the two proteins takes place and both mechanisms are operative. Integrins, once engaged by the proper ligand, can activate hERG1 channels which, in turn, modulate integrin function.

Our first reports in this field showed that, in mouse[46] and human[47] neuroblastoma cells, hERG1 activation was one of the earliest integrin-mediated "outside-to-in" signals. In these cells, a few minutes after cell contact with proteins of the extracellular matrix (ECM), fibronectin (FN)[46] or laminin (LM),[47] a sustained increase in hERG1 current density occurred (see Fig. 2). Such increase was mediated by the β1 integrin engagement. At difference from mouse neuroblastoma

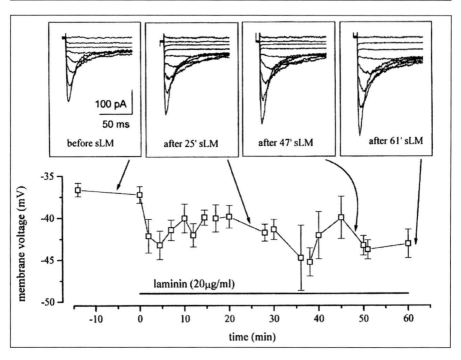

Figure 2. hERG1 current increase in human neuroblastoma cells SH-SY5Y, after addition of soluble Laminin (sLM). Currents were recorded through perforated patch. Pictures are from Arcangeli A et al, 1996 (ref. 46) with permission.

cells, in which hERG1 activation by FN was always accompanied by hyperpolarization, in human neuroblastoma cells this effect was only observed when LM was added in soluble form. On the contrary, cell adhesion onto substrate-bound LM activated both hERG1 and stretch activated depolarizing channels, which produced little net effect on V_m.[47] Once again, the effect of soluble and substrate-bound LM was found to depend on β1 integrin subunit. The specificity of β1 in the integrin-mediated activation of hERG1 was further demonstrated in a human preosteoclastic leukemia cell line (FLG 29.1),[48] as well as in HEK 293 stably expressing the *herg1* encoding cDNA.[49] In particular, in FLG 29.1 cells, different antibodies activating either α or β integrin subunits were tested, but only those directed to β1 activated hERG1. Hence, neither α subunits, nor β subunits other than β1, are involved in the hERG1 activation in tumor cells. In all of these experimental systems, integrin engagement produced an increase in hERG1 current density, without any significant variation of the hERG1 protein surface expression. Therefore, β1 must somehow affect hERG1 gating, most probably through an increase of channel open probability, as we have shown for the integrin activation of Ca^{2+}-dependent K^+ channels in erythroleukemia cells. How can this occur? Studies on the cardiac hERG1 channel have shown a complex interplay between PKA[50] and PKC[51] in channel regulation. Other mechanisms apparently take place in microglial cells, where a c-Src-dependent tyrosine phosphorylation of the channel protein affect hERG1 activity[52] and in TRH sensitive pituitary cells. In these cells, hERG channels are differentially regulated by small GTPases, so that RhoA inhibits whereas Rac produces stimulation.[53] Interestingly, the regulatory effect of TRH on hERG1 is mainly caused by modulation of the hERG1B subunit.[54] Similar mechanisms could also operate in the case of integrin-dependent control, since most of the above regulatory proteins are often recruited by integrin activation.[16] We have shown, for example, that a pertussis toxin-sensitive G protein mediates the integrin-dependent hERG1 activation in neuroblastoma and leukemia cells.[46-48] The triggering mechanism appears to require a physical interaction between β1 and the channel, although it is still unclear whether protein-protein interaction is sufficient to stimulate hERG1 activation or the macromolecular complex recruits or activates further cytosolic elements that in turn affect the channels ativity. This situation is similar to that described for the 14-3-3 adaptor protein, which is known to regulate hERG1 by forming molecular complexes with the channel protein.[50,52]

Integrins and hERG1 Channels form a Macromolecular Complex

The assembly of integrins with ion channels is not a novelty. Kv 1.3 channels and the β1 integrin physically interact in T-lymphocytes and this leads to the activation of integrin adhesive properties and subsequent cell migration.[55] The physical link between Kv 1.3 channels and β1 integrins has also been described in melanoma cells.[56]

A physical association also occurs between the β1 integrin subunit and the hERG1 channel, as witnessed by the fact that the two proteins can be co-immunoprecipitated from membrane protein extracts of different cancer cells.[28,49,57,58] The biochemical characteristics of the β1/hERG1 complex was studied in detail in a reconstituted system, represented by HEK 293 cells stably transfected with the *herg1* cDNA.[49] The two proteins co-immunoprecipitated in basal culture conditions, i.e., in the presence of serum. However, the formation of the β1/hERG1 complex was further stimulated by either cell adhesion onto FN or addition of the anti β1 activating antibody to suspended cells. Hence, assembly of the complex is independent from cell adhesion but strictly dependent on β1 activation. The formation of the complex started after 15 min of integrin stimulation and reached its maximal activation at 30 min. At that time, the complex also comprised Caveolin-1, suggesting its targeting to caveolae/lipid rafts. It is worth noting that the time course of complex formation fits well with that of hERG1 current activation (see Fig. 2).

Further indications on the molecular characteristics of the complex came from experiments performed on HEK 293 transiently expressing hERG1B, or another channel of the same family, EAG. In both cases, no co-immunoprecipitation of the expressed channel with β1 occurred. The lack of co-immunoprecipiation of β1 with hERG1B suggests that the hERG1 N-terminus is necessary for the membrane complex formation. However, the intracellular PAS domain is unlikely to be relevant, since EAG channels possess a PAS domain identical to the hERG1's and still do not form a complex with β1 integrin. Moreover, because the N-terminus of hERG1 is located intracellularly, some corresponding intracellular domain of the integrin subunit should be envisaged as the partner domain. The most likely candidate is the short intracellular C-terminus of β1 integrin, although we cannot exclude the involvement of intramembrane domain(s). Whatever the mechanism, recent FRET experiments confirmed the direct interaction between these two proteins. As described in Chapter 4, the FRET technique is one of the most suitable methods to study direct interactions between proteins. We have adapted this method to study the β1 integrin and hERG1, using recombinant fluorescent proteins transfected into HEK 293 cells. Images were analyzed with a TIRFM apparatus, to detect plasma membrane proteins only (see Chapter 4 for details). We showed the occurrence of energy transfer between the two molecules in HEK 293 cells in basal conditions, i.e., in the presence of serum. Besides supporting the findings obtained with indirect biochemical methods, these results also demonstrates that the two proteins interact directly, since the intermolecular distance turned out to be lower than 10 nm (Masi A., personal communication).

Using the same experimental model and employing biochemical methods, we also showed that the β1/hERG1 complex, once formed and translocated into caveolae/lipid rafts, recruits one of the most relevant downstream effectors of integrin activation, i.e. the cytoplasmic tyrosine kinase FAK. This occurs 60 min after integrin engagement and is dependent on hERG1 channel activity, being impaired by specific hERG1 blockers. These, however, do not affect the formation of the β1/hERG1 complex. With a similar time course and dependence on hERG1 channel activity, the small GTPase Rac1 is also recruited in the β1/hERG1 complex. We have obtained analogous results in colorectal cancer cells (Masi A., personal communication) and conclude that, in epithelial cells, integrin activation by proper ligands lead to association with hERG1. The multiprotein complex translocates to caveolae/lipid rafts, where hERG1 is activated. Subsequently, activated channels promote the recruitment, into plasma membrane microdomains, of different signaling proteins, like FAK and Rac1.

In other experimental systems, the β1/hERG1 complex comprises different plasma membrane proteins. For example, in acute myeloid leukemia (AML), as well as in human cytokine-stimulated hemopoietic progenitor cells, the complex has an adjunctive partner represented by the VEGF receptor 1 (Flt-1).[28] In this case, the membrane complex almost exclusively involves the hERG1B isoform, which, as mentioned above, is highly expressed in leukemia cells. Why hERG1B does not co-immunoprecipitate with the β1 integrin in transfected HEK 293 cells while it does in AML cells? We showed that, in AML cells, Flt-1 and hERG1B co-immunoprecipitate also in basal conditions, without VEGF-A addition.[28] In these conditions, the β1 integrin is absent from the complex, whereas it is promptly recruited after integrin stimulation. Hence, in AML cells, it is possible that β1 mostly interacts with Flt-1, as occurs in other experimental models,[59] instead of hERG1B (see Fig. 3). The latter, on the contrary, could bind to Flt-1, probably through a protein domain different from that used by hERG1 when associating with β1, perhaps an intra- or transmembrane domain.

Another multiprotein complex formed by hERG1 with membrane receptors was observed in acute B lymphoblastic leukemias (B-ALL).[58] Here again a tri-molecular complex occurs which involves the β$_1$ integrin subunit and the chemokine receptor CXCR4, besides hERG1. CXCR4 is a seven transmembrane domain chemokine receptor, activated by the stromal-derived-factor 1 (SDF-1). The complex turned out to be tri-molecular also in starved cells, in this case. In fact, hERG1 co-immunoprecipitates with both β1 and CXCR4, in the absence on any stimulation (Pillozzi S., personal communication). Based on these data, we hypothesize that, in B-ALL cells, the integrin behaves as the central member of the complex, interacting with both the chemokine receptor, as documented in other systems[60] and the ion channel. If this double interaction involves different domains of the integrin molecule, as outlined in the picture in Figure 3, awaits demonstration.

Altogether it emerges that, when forming a macromolecular complex with hERG1 channels, the partner membrane proteins form signaling platforms in which further proteins and/or second messengers can be concentrated. These platforms constitute signaling sites that trigger and sustain intracellular messages (see below).

Effects of hERG1 Activation on Integrin Function and Signaling

Which is the significance of the integrin/hERG1 interaction? Has the integrin-mediated hERG1 channel activation any relevance in cellular function? Our early data indicated that the integrin-dependent activation of hERG1 channels was relevant in the modulation of cell differentiation, in both neuroblastoma and pre-osteoclastic leukemia cells. In fact, blocking hERG1 almost abolished neurite emission induced, in neuroblastoma cells, by adhesion onto FN or LM.[46,47] In the pre-osteoclastic leukemia model, inhibiting the FN-induced hERG1 activation dramatically impaired the acquisition of the osteoclast phenotype typically triggered by cell adhesion. In these cells, differentiation is accompanied by expression of αvβ3 integrin.[48] Therefore, an interesting double cross talk between integrins and hERG1 channels emerges: while the β1 integrin activates hERG1, the activated channels increase the membrane expression of β3, a different integrin subunit.

In AML cells, the β1/hERG1/Flt-1 complex regulates different biological phenomena, i.e., leukemia cell proliferation and migration. Both processes were in fact inhibited, in vitro, when hERG1 channel activity was specifically blocked.[28] In childhood B-ALL, the β1/hERG1/CXCR4 complex has the function of overcoming drug resistance.[58] It is worth recalling that, in childhood B-ALL, the bone marrow microenvironment provides a "sanctuary" in which subpopulations of leukemia cells can evade chemotherapy-induced death and acquire a drug-resistant phenotype. The bone marrow-mediated protection involves a complex interplay between stroma-produced cyto- and chemokines, as well as adhesion molecules and their receptors on leukemia cells.[61,62] Hence, when B-ALL cell lines are cultured on human bone marrow stromal cells, the apoptotic effect

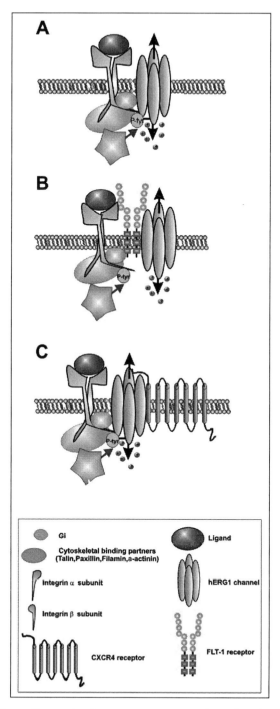

Figure 3. Mechanisms of interaction between integrins, ion channels and GF(growth factor) or chemokine receptors. Model for the hERG1 regulated macromolecular complexes: A) hERG1/β1 complex; B) hERG1/FLT-1/β1 complex and C) CXCR4/hERG1/β1 complex.

of chemotherapic drugs like doxorubicin, prednisone, vincristin and methotraxate are strongly inhibited. In these conditions, the addition of specific hERG1 blockers bypasses the resistance to such drugs, promptly restoring a significant apoptosis in leukemia cells (Pillozzi et al, unpublished results). Finally, in colorectal cancer, the β1/hERG1/FAK complex regulates the cell invasiveness triggered by adhesion onto an integrin-dependent matrix, i.e., Matrigel. The process is strictly dependent on both hERG1 expression level and activity.[9]

How can hERG1 channels, once activated and bound to integrins, modulate such a variety of cellular functions? The activity of hERG1 channels could control both the adhesive and signaling functions of integrins. For instance, HEK 293 cells overexpressing hERG1 display a stimulated cell spreading onto FN, compared to the controls.[49] Moreover, hERG1, when complexed with integrins, modulates integrin-dependent signaling. In fact, not only FAK and Rac-1 co-immunoprecipitate with hERG1 upon adhesion onto FN, but such interaction is necessary for the subsequent tyrosine phosphorylation (p-tyr) of FAK and for Rac-1 switch on.[49] The β1/hERG1/Flt-1 complex in AML cells is necessary for Flt-1 p-tyr and the activation of downstream signaling (MAPK and PI3K/pAkt activation). hERG1 channel activity was necessary for both the modulation of intracellular signaling and the triggering of biological effects, i.e., cell survival (MAPK) and cell migration (PI3K/pAKT).[28] The β1/hERG1/CXCR4 complex in B-ALL cells triggers the activation of both MAPK and PI3K/pAKT intracellular pathways. The specific block of hERG1 channel activity inhibits both of the pathways, underlining again the hERG1 role as a molecular device that regulates integrin- and chemokine receptors-dependent signaling (Pillozzi S., personal communication).

Conclusion

On the whole, three types of integrin/hERG1 channel complexes have been identified so far:
1. a β1/hERG1/FAK_Rac-1 complex, prevalently expressed in epithelial cells and mainly devoted to the regulation of cell invasiveness;
2. a β1/hERG1/Flt-1, expressed in myeloid leukemia cells and devoted to the regulation of cell proliferation and invasion;
3. a β1/hERG1/CXCR4 complex, expressed in lymphoid leukemia cells and responsible for mediating chemoresistance.

The first type of complex functions presumably because it interferes with FAK- and Rac-1-centred signaling, hence linking the plasma membrane to the cytoskeleton and in turn to the cell motility machinery; the other complexes mainly act by modulating signaling triggered by GF or chemokine receptors, interfering with pathways that further overlap with those triggered by integrins. In any case, the presence and activity of the channel protein inside the complex is determinant in regulating signaling activity of the entire complex, as witnessed by the use of channel blockers. These effects of the channel protein could be more or less dependent on the classic effects of hERG1 on V_m, or could occur through conformational coupling between the channel and the interacting proteins. This latter effect could more or less depend on ion fluxes, depending on whether the intracellular modulatory domains are conformationally associated or not with the gating process (see above). At the present time it is not possible to distinguish between these two possibilities. As far as we are aware, all the known hERG1 inhibitors block the ion conduction pathway. Therefore, this problem must be approached by different techniques by using nonconductive hERG1 mutants.

Finally, these and other results from different sources convey the hypothesis that drugs acting on ion channels could have therapeutic value in cancer treatment. Recent evidence suggests that, in certain tumors, application of channel inhibitors does in fact impair cell growth both in vitro and in vivo.[2] A major objection to such a pharmacological approach is the presence of serious side effects, particularly cardiac arrhythmias. This flaw is now being overcome by different approaches, for example the identification of non-arrhythmogenic compounds or calibration of treatment by exploitation of drug selectivity for specific channel states.[2] Finally, a novel therapeutic approach could be developed by unlocking ion channels from multiprotein membrane signaling complexes, as suggested by work on hERG1. Once the functional epitopes involved in hERG1 binding with its partners have been determined, penetrating peptides, capable of competing with these epitopes could be used to unlock the membrane complexes.

Acknowledgments

This work has been supported by grants from the Associazione Italiana per la Ricerca sul Cancro (AIRC), Association for International Cancer Research (AICR), Ministero dell'Universtá e della Ricerca Scientifica e technologica (PRIN 2005), Associazione Genitori Noi per Voi and Ente Cassa di Risparmio di Firenze to AA.

References

1. De Vita V, Hellmann S, Rosenberg S. Cancer. Principles and practice of oncology, Lippincott Williams and Wilkins: New York 2008.
2. Arcangeli A, Crociani O, Lastraioli E et al. Targeting ion channels in cancer: a novel frontier in antineoplastic therapy. Curr Med Chem 2009; 16: 66-93.
3. Fraser SP, Pardo LA. Ion channels: functional expression and therapeutic potential in cancer. Colloquium on Ion Channels and Cancer. EMBO Rep 2008; 9:512-515.
4. Wonderlin WF, Strobl JS. Potassium channels, proliferation and G1 progression. J Membr Biol 1996; 154:91-107.
5. Pardo LA. Voltage-gated potassium channels in cell proliferation. Physiology (Bethesda) 2004; 19:285-292.
6. Arcangeli A, Becchetti A. Ion channels and the cell cycle. In: D. Janigro, ed. The Cell Cycle in the Nervous Central System. Hartford:Humana Press, 2006.
7. Diss JK, Fraser SP, Djamgoz MB. Voltage-gated Na$^+$ channels: multiplicity of expression, plasticity, functional implications and pathophysiological aspects. Eur Biophys J 2004; 33:180-193.
8. Fraser SP, Diss JK, Chioni AM et al. Voltage-gated sodium channel expression and potentiation of human breast cancer metastasis. Clin Cancer Res 2005; 11:5381-5389.
9. Lastraioli E, Guasti L, Crociani O et al. Herg1 gene and HERG1 protein are overexpressed in colorectal cancers and regulate cell invasion of tumor cells. Cancer Res 2004; 64:606-611.
10. Olsen ML, Schade S, Lyons SA et al. Expression of voltage-gated chloride channels in human glioma cells. J Neurosci 2003; 23:5572-5582.
11. Olsen ML, Weaver AK, Ritch PS et al. Modulation of glioma BK channels via erbB2. J Neurosci Res 2005; 81:179-189.
12. Sontheimer H. An unexpected role for ion channels in brain tumor metastasis. Experimental biology and medicine 2008; 233:779-791.
13. Beeton C, Wulff H, Standifer NE et al. Kv1.3 channels are a therapeutic target for T-cell-mediated autoimmune diseases. Proc Natl Acad Sci USA 2006; 103:17414-17419.
14. Mamelak AN, Rosenfeld S, Bucholz R et al. Phase I single-dose study of intracavitary-administered iodine-131-TM-601 in adults with recurrent high-grade glioma. J Clin Oncol 2006; 24:3644-3650.
15. Hegle AP, Marble DD, Wilson GF. A voltage-driven switch for ion-independent signaling by ether-à-go-go K$^+$ channels. Proc Natl Acad Sci USA 2006; 103:2886-2891.
16. Arcangeli A, Becchetti A. Complex functional interaction between integrin receptors and ion channels. Trends Cell Biol 2006; 16:631-639.
17. Arcangeli A. Expression and role of hERG channels in cancer cells. Novartis Found Symp 2005; 266:225-232.
18. Warmke JW, Ganetzky B. A family of potassium channel genes related to eag in Drosophila and mammals. Proc Natl Acad Sci USA 1994; 91(8):3438-3442.
19. Sanguinetti MC, Jiang C, Curran ME et al. A mechanistic link between an inherited and an acquired cardiac arrhythmia: HERG encodes the IKr potassium channel. Cell 1995; 81:299-307.
20. Bauer CK, Schwarz JR. Physiology of EAG K$^+$ channels. J Membr Biol 2001; 182:1-15.
21. Crociani O, Cherubini A, Piccini E et al. Erg gene(s) expression during development of the nervous and muscular system of quail embryos. Mech Dev 2000; 95:239-243.
22. Polvani S, Masi A, Pillozzi S et al. Developmentally regulated expression of the mouse homologues of the potassium channel encoding genes m-erg1, m-erg2 and m-erg3. Gene Expr Patterns 2003; 3:767-776.
23. Sanguinetti MC, Tristani-Firouzi M. HERG potassium channels and cardiac arrhythmia. Nature 2006; 440:463-469.
24. Keating MT. Genetic approaches to cardiovascular disease. Supravalvular aortic stenosis, Williams syndrome and long-QT syndrome. Circulation 1995; 92:142-147.
25. Crociani O, Guasti L, Balzi M et al. Cell cycle-dependent expression of HERG1 and HERG1B isoforms in tumor cells. J Biol Chem 2003; 278: 2947-2955.

26. Jones EM, Roti Roti EC, Wang J et al. Cardiac IKr channels minimally comprise hERG 1a and 1b subunits. J Biol Chem 2004; 279:44690-44694.
27. Guasti L, Crociani O, Redaelli E et al. Identification of a posttranslational mechanism for the regulation of hERG1 K+ channels expression and hERG1 current density in tumor cells. Mol Cell Biol 2008; 28:5043-5060.
28. Pillozzi S, Brizzi MF, Bernabei PA. VEGFR-1 (FLT-1), beta1 integrin and hERG K+ channel for a macromolecular signaling complex in acute myeloid leukemia: role in cell migration and clinical outcome. Blood 2007; 110:1238-1250.
29. Kupershmidt S, Snyders DJ, Raes A et al. A K+ channel splice variant common in human heart lacks a C-terminal domain required for expression of rapidly activating delayed rectifier current. J Biol Chem 1998; 273:27231-27235.
30. Chiesa N, Rosati B, Arcangeli A et al. A novel role for HERG K+ channels: spike-frequency adaptation. J Physiol 1997; 501:313-318.
31. Sacco T, De Luca A, Tempia F. Properties and expression of Kv3 channels in cerebellar Purkinje cells. Mol Cell Neurosi 2006; 33:170-179.
32. Furlan F, Taccola G, Grandolfo M et al. ERG conductance expression modulates the excitability of ventral horn GABAergic interneurons that control rhythmic oscillations in the developing mouse spinal cord. J Neurosci 2007; 27:919-928.
33. Arcangeli A, Bianchi L, Becchetti A et al. A novel inward-rectifying K+ current with a cell-cycle dependence governs the resting potential of mammalian neuroblastoma cells. J Physiol 1995; 489:455-471.
34. Binggeli R, Weinstein RCJ. Membrane potentials and sodium channels: hypotheses for growth regulation and cancer formation based on changes in sodium channels and gap junctions. Theor Biol 1986; 123:377-401.
35. Schönherr R, Rosati B, Hehl S et al. Functional role of the slow activation property of ERG K+ channels. Eur J Neurosci 1999; 11:753-760.
36. Pillozzi S, Brizzi MF, Balzi M et al. HERG potassium channels are constitutively expressed in primary human acute myeloid leukemias and regulate cell proliferation of normal and leukemic hemopoietic progenitors. Leukemia 2002; 16:1791-1798.
37. Smith GA, Tsui H, Newell EW et al. Functional up-regulation of HERG K+ channels in neoplastic hematopoietic cells. J Biol Chem 2002; 277:18528-18534.
38. Shao X, Wu K, Hao Z et al. The potent inhibitory effects of cisapride, a specific blocker for human ether-A-Go-Go-Related gene (HERG) channel, on gastric cancer cells. Cancer Biol Ther 2005; 4:295-301.
39. Lastraioli E, Gasperi Campani F, Taddei A et al. On behalf of GIRCG "hERG1 channels are overexpressed in human gastric cancer and their activity regulates cell proliferation: a novel prognostic and therapeutic target?" In: Proceedings of the 6th International Gastric Cancer Congress IGCC, Yokohama (Japan) 2005.
40. Shao X, Wu K, Guo X et al. Expression and significance of HERG protein in gastric cancer. Cancer Biol Ther 2008; 7:45-50.
41. Witchel HJ, Hancox JC. Familial and acquired long qt syndrome and the cardiac rapid delayed rectifier potassium current. Clin Exp Pharmacol Physiol 2000; 27:753-766.
42. Shah RR. Drug-induced QT interval prolongation—regulatory guidance and perspectives on hERG channel studies. Novartis Found Symp 2005; 266:251-80.
43. Masi A, Becchetti A, Restano-Cassulini R et al. HERG1 channels are overexpressed in glioblastoma multiforme and modulate VEGF secretion in glioblastoma cell lines. Br J Cancer 2005; 93:781-92.
44. Lastraioli E, Taddei A, Messerini L et al. HERG1 channels in human esophagus: evidence for their aberrant expression in the malignant progression of Barrett's esophagus. J Cell Physiol 2006; 209:398-404.
45. Lin H, Xiao J, Luo X et al. Overexpression HERG K+ channel gene mediates cell-growth signals on activation of oncoproteins SP1 and NF-kappaB and inactivation of tumor suppressor Nkx3.1. J Cell Physiol 2007; 212:137-147.
46. Arcangeli A, Becchetti A, Mannini A et al. Integrin-mediated neurite outgrowth in neuroblastoma cells depends on the activation of potassium channels. J Cell Biol 1993; 122:113-1143.
47. Arcangeli A, Faravelli L, Bianchi L et al. Soluble or bound laminin elicit in human neuroblastoma cells short- or long-term potentiation of a K+ inwardly rectifying current: relevance to neuritogenesis. Cell Adhes Commun 1996; 4:369-385.
48. Hofmann G, Bernabei PA, Crociani O et al. HERG K+ channels activation during beta(1) integrin-mediated adhesion to fibronectin induces an up-regulation of alpha(v)beta(3) integrin in the preosteoclastic leukemia cell line FLG 29.1. J Biol Chem 2001; 276:4923-4931.

49. Cherubini A, Hofmann G, Pillozzi S et al. Human ether-a-go-go-related gene 1 channels are physically linked to beta1 integrins and modulate adhesion-dependent signaling. Mol Biol Cell 2005; 16:2972-2983.
50. Kagan A, McDonald TV. Dynamic control of hERG/I(Kr) by PKA-mediated interactions with 14-3-3. Novartis Found Symp 2005; 266:75-89.
51. Bian JS, McDonald TV. Phosphatidylinositol 4,5-bisphosphate interactions with the HERG K(+) channel. Pflugers Arch 2007; 455:105-113.
52. Cayabyab FS, Tsui FW, Schlichter LC. Modulation of the ERG K$^+$ current by the tyrosine phosphatase, SHP-1. J Biol Chem 2002; 277:48130-48138.
53. Miranda P, Giráldez T, de la Peña P et al. Specificity of TRH receptor coupling to G-proteins for regulation of ERG K$^+$ channels in GH3 rat anterior pituitary cells. J Physiol 2005; 566:717-736.
54. Kirchberger NM, Wulfsen I, Schwarz JR et al. Effects of TRH on heteromeric rat erg1a/1b K$^+$ channels are dominated by the rerg1b subunit. J Physiol 2006; 571:27-42.
55. Levite M, Cahalon L, Peretz A et al. Extracellular K$^+$ and opening of voltage-gated potassium channels activate T-cell integrin function: physical and functional association between Kv1.3 channels and beta1 integrins. J Exp Med 2000; 191:1167-1176.
56. Artym VV, Petty HR. Molecular proximity of Kv1.3 voltage-gated potassium channels and beta(1)-integrins on the plasma membrane of melanoma cells: effects of cell adherence and channel blockers. J Gen Physiol 2002; 120:29-37.
57. Cherubini A, Pillozzi S, Hofmann G et al. HERG K$^+$ channels and beta1 integrins interact through the assembly of a macromolecular complex. Ann N Y Acad Sci 2002; 973:559-561.
58. Pillozzi S, Accordi B, Veltroni M et al. Blood (ASH Annual Meeting Abstracts) 2007; 110:877.
59. Orecchia A, Lacal PM, Schietroma C et al. Vascular endothelial growth factor receptor-1 is deposited in the extracellular matrix by endothelial cells and is a ligand for the α5β1 integrin. J Cell Sci 2003; 116:3479–3489.
60. Ngo HT, Leleu X, Lee J et al. SDF-1/CXCR4 and VLA-4 interaction regulates homing in Waldenstrom macroglobulinemia. Blood 2008; 112:150-158.
61. Garrido SM, Appelbaum FR, Willman CL et al. Acute myeloid leukemia cells are protected from spontaneous and drug-induced apoptosis by direct contact with a human bone marrow stromal cell line (HS-5). Exp Hematol 2001; 29:448-457.
62. Tabe Y, Jin L, Tsutsumi-Ishii Y et al. Activation of integrin-linked kinase is a critical prosurvival pathway induced in leukemic cells by bone marrow-derived stromal cells. Cancer Res 2007; 67:684-694.

CHAPTER 7

Coordinated Regulation of Vascular Ca²⁺ and K⁺ Channels by Integrin Signaling

Peichun Gui, Jun-Tzu Chao, Xin Wu, Yan Yang, George E. Davis and Michael J. Davis*

Abstract

A role for integrins in mechanotransduction has been suggested because these molecules form an important mechanical link between the extracellular matrix (ECM) and the cytoskeleton. An example of mechanotransduction in blood vessels is the myogenic response—the rapid and maintained constriction of arterioles in response to pressure elevation. L-type calcium channels and large-conductance, calcium-activated potassium (BK) channels are known to play important roles in the myogenic response and in the maintenance of myogenic (pressure-induced) vascular tone. Our recent studies on isolated, cannulated arterioles and freshly-dispersed arteriolar smooth muscle cells show that both L-type calcium channels (Ca$_v$1.2) and BK channels are regulated by α5β1 integrin activation. α5β1 integrin interacts with the ECM protein fibronectin, which is distributed in basement membrane and interstitial matrices surrounding smooth muscle cells within the arteriolar wall. Truncation and site-directed mutagenesis strategies reveal that regulation of Ca$_v$1.2 by α5β1 integrin requires phosphorylation of the channel α$_{1C}$ subunit at C-terminal residues Ser-1901 and Tyr-2122. Likewise, BK channel potentiation by α5β1 integrin activation requires c-Src phosphorylation of the channel α-subunit at residue Tyr-766. Thus, both L-type calcium channels and BK channels can be regulated coordinately through integrin-linked phosphorylation cascades involving c-Src. We propose that these two channels are under constitutive control by α5β1 integrin-fibronectin interactions in the vessel wall such that the balance of their activity determines myogenic tone and the vascular response to vessel wall injury/remodeling.

Introduction

Integrins are a large family of cell surface receptors that provide for adhesion of cells to the extracellular matrix (ECM). In addition, integrins act as a membrane coupling and assembly point for a wide variety of cytoskeletal and cell signaling components.[1-4] As such, integrins are strategically positioned to structurally and mechanically integrate the extracellular and intracellular environments along an "ECM-integrin-cytoskeletal axis".[5,6] Integrins consist of one α and one β subunit joined noncovalently. At least 10 of the more than 22 known integrin subunit combinations have been identified in vascular smooth muscle (VSM): α1β1, α2β1, α3β1, α4β1, α5β1, α7β1, α8β1, α9β1, αvβ3, and α6β4.[7] The predominance of α1β1, α3β1, α5β1, αvβ1 and αvβ3 integrins in VSM suggests there are extensive interactions with their respective ECM ligands—collagen I, collagen IV, laminin and fibronectin (FN)—in the basement membrane and interstitial matrix.[7] Integrins

*Corresponding Author: Michael J. Davis—Dept. Medical Pharmacology and Physiology, University of Missouri School of Medicine, 1 Hospital Dr., Rm. M451, Columbia, Missouri 65212, USA. Email: davismj@health.missouri.edu

Integrins and Ion Channels: Molecular Complexes and Signaling, edited by Andrea Becchetti and Annarosa Arcangeli. ©2010 Landes Bioscience and Springer Science+Business Media.

have been proposed to be key elements in mechanosensation/transduction processes, examples of which include the responses of blood vessels to shear stress and transmural pressure.[8,9] Thus, integrin-mediated signaling in VSM and endothelium may be important for controlling blood flow by myogenic and flow-dependent responses, where integrins are part of a tension-sensing mechanism in the vascular wall.[10-17] Because strong pharmacological evidence implicates Ca^{2+} and K^+ channels in these vascular responses,[18-20] we tested the hypothesis that ion channels in VSM and endothelium were regulated by ECM-integrin interactions.

Regulation of L-Type Calcium Channels by Integrin Activation

The L-type calcium (Ca_L) channel is the major Ca^{2+}-entry pathway in VSM and is critical for myogenic constriction and the maintenance of myogenic tone. Isolated, cannulated arterioles from skeletal muscle develop spontaneous, pressure-dependent tone, constricting to ~30-50% of maximal passive diameter;[11] this tone is modulated by both pressure changes and agonists. Interestingly, myogenic tone is also acutely altered by the extraluminal application of integrin ligands such as RGD (arginine-glycine-aspartic acid) peptide, cyclic RGD (cRGD) peptide,[11] as well as fibronectin fragments (unpublished observations) and digested collagen fragments.[12] These observations led us to investigate whether VSM ion channels were involved in mediating the responses to integrin ligands. In initial, whole-cell patch clamp recordings from cremaster arteriolar myocytes, we observed that the application of soluble FN caused acute inhibition of an inward current (Fig 1). Under these recording conditions, inward Ca_L currents are typically superimposed on much larger, outward K^+ currents. Indeed, we routinely observed that FN and other soluble integrin ligands, such as RGD-containing peptides, primarily inhibited the net current at voltages where the contribution of Ca_L would be greatest. In addition, the arteriolar dilation to cRGD

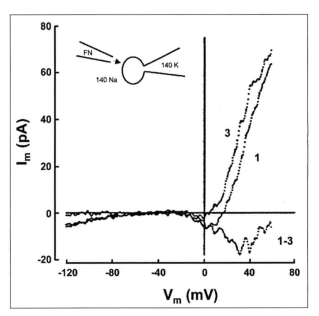

Figure 1. Current-voltage (I-V) relationship of whole-cell current in a VSM cell under conditions where both L-type Ca^{2+} channels and K^+ channels are active. Trace 1 represents the current evoked by a voltage ramp from −120 to +80 mV under control (unstimulated) conditions. Trace 3 was obtained after the addition of soluble FN fragment (120 kD). Trace 1-3 is the difference current, showing that the major effect of soluble FN in this cell is to inhibit a small inward current that peaked at +30 mV. Bath, 140 mM Na^+ physiological saline solution; Pipette, physiological saline solution with equimolar substitution of K^+ for Na^+.

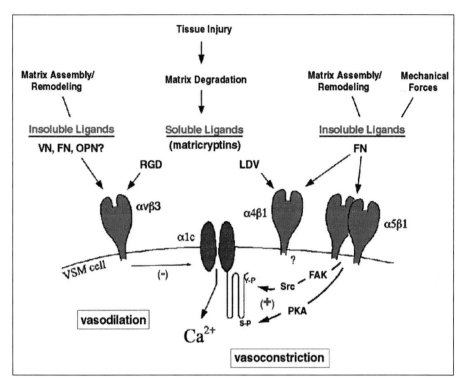

Figure 2. Diagram summarizing the known signaling pathways between αvβ3, α4β1 and α5β1 integrins and the L-type Ca²⁺ channel in VSM. Also illustrated are the hypothesized mechanisms for physiological and pathological activation of integrin-channel signaling mechanisms, including mechanical force application, chronic remodeling of the vessel wall/matrix and matrix degradation. Modified from Davis M. et al. 2002; 36:41-66;[59] with permission.

peptide is preceded by a decrease in VSM $[Ca^{2+}]_i$, suggesting that the peptide acts by interfering with a calcium entry mechanism.[21] For these reasons we concentrated our subsequent efforts on understanding the effects of integrin ligands on VSM Ca_L channels.

To summarize several years of work, we find that Ca_L channels are regulated by at least three different VSM integrins (Fig. 2). Whole-cell patch-clamp recordings from single, freshly-dissociated arteriolar myocytes showed that both soluble and insoluble ligands of αvβ3 integrin (the vitronectin receptor), including RGD, cRGD, vitronectin and fibronectin fragments, acutely inhibited Ca_L current when it was measured in isolation from larger whole-cell K⁺ currents.[22] In contrast, Ca_L current was potentiated by ligands of α5β1 integrin, but only insoluble α5β1 integrin ligands; for example, soluble α5β1 integrin antibody failed to modulate current unless a secondary antibody was subsequently applied to aggregate the integrin.[22] Collectively, the requirement for an insoluble α5β1 integrin ligand to modulate channel function is consistent with the observations of many other laboratories that only multivalent integrin ligands can induce integrin ligation, aggregation, redistribution/recruitment of focal adhesion proteins and subsequent activation of signaling cascades involving nonreceptor tyrosine kinases.[23] Consistent with this conclusion was our observation that the effect of insoluble α5β1 ligands on Ca_L current was prevented by the nonspecific tyrosine kinase inhibitors genistein, piceatannol, or by the Src-family kinase inhibitor, PP2.[24] Furthermore, dialysis of VSM cells through the patch pipettes with an antibody to c-Src largely prevented Ca_L current potentiation following α5β1 integrin activation. Conversely, phosphatase inhibition increased both basal Ca_L current and the magnitude of Ca_L current potentiated by α5β1 integrin activation.[24]

With regard to other integrins, we have been unable to see any effect of α1β1, α2β1, or α3β1 integrin ligands on VSM Ca_L current (unpublished observations), which suggests that only certain integrins are coupled to VSM ion channel signaling. However, soluble ligands of α4β1 integrin, such as Leu-Asp-Val (LDV) peptide, potentiate VSM Ca_L current similar to the effect of α5β1 integrin activation and this potentiation is also associated with *Src* family tyrosine kinase activation.[17] The enhancement in current is similar in time course, but lower in magnitude, to that seen in response to multivalent α5β1 integrin ligands.[22]

Collectively, these observations are consistent with data from other smooth muscle preparations in which Ca^{2+} current was observed to increase in response to intracellular application of constitutively active Src kinase[25] or c-Src activating peptide and experiments in which Ca_L current was inhibited by a c-Src monoclonal antibody.[26,27] Additionally, platelet-derived growth factor, which stimulates tyrosine phosphorylation of multiple smooth muscle proteins, enhances Ca_L current in smooth muscle[28] and increases tyrosine phosphorylation of the pore-forming channel subunit $α_{1C}$ ($Ca_v1.2b$).[27] Thus, links between tyrosine phosphorylation and Ca_L channel regulation in smooth muscle are well established.

Our studies also indicate that other Ca_L isoform besides VSM Ca_L ($Ca_v1.2b$) can be potentiated by α5β1 activation (Fig. 3). Using a heterologous expression system lacking endogenous $Ca_v1.2$ channels (HEK 293 cells), the expression of either $Ca_v1.2b$ or $Ca_v1.2c$ (neuronal) channels resulted in robust and stable voltage-gated Ca_L currents that were potentiated ~2-fold in response to α5β1 integrin activation, i.e., after application of α5β1 integrin antibody. Only the pore-forming $α_{1C}$ channel subunit is critical for these responses since they could be reproduced in the absence of the appropriate β and $α_2$-δ accessory channel subunits. We have also observed that $Ca_v1.2a$ (the cardiac isoform) is potentiated by α5β1 integrin activation,[29] which is consistent with the observations by at least one other group that cardiac Ca_L currents are modulated by the ECM.[30,31]

We subsequently applied truncation and site-directed mutagenesis strategies to cloned $Ca_v1.2c$ channels to more definitively probe the mechanism of channel regulation by integrin activation. Our studies revealed that regulation of the channel by α5β1 integrin requires phosphorylation of C-terminal residues Ser-1901 and Tyr-2122 on the pore-forming $α_{1C}$ channel subunit.[32] These sites are known to be phosphorylated by PKA and c-Src, respectively and are conserved between rat neuronal and rat smooth muscle $Ca_v1.2$ isoforms (Fig. 4). Kinase assays performed on immunoprecipitated $Ca_v1.2$ channels are consistent with phosphorylation of the same two residues by PKA and c-Src. Following α5β1 integrin activation, native Ca_L channels in freshly isolated VSM cells from rat skeletal muscle arterioles exhibit potentiation that is completely blocked by selective and combined PKA and c-Src inhibition.[32]

Recently, we also examined the potential spatial interactions between the Ca_L channel and α5β1 integrin. Immunoprecipitation protocols reveal that α5 and β1 integrins co-associate with wild-type $Ca_v1.2c$ in cells plated on fibronectin but not on poly-l-lysine (unpublished observations), suggesting a requirement for α5β1 integrin engagement and clustering. The degree of Ca_L and α5β1 integrin co-association is reduced in a $Ca_v1.2$ mutant lacking the distal C-terminus and in a $Ca_v1.2$ mutant in which only the C-terminal proline-rich domain (1948-1973) is deleted.[33] Thus, the C-terminus of the Ca_L channel may be critical for interaction with α5β1 integrin or an associated focal adhesion protein.

Collectively, these findings suggest that PKA, c-Src and possibly other tyrosine kinases colocalize with Ca_L channels to facilitate regulation by integrin engagement/disengagement. Furthermore, the common effect of α5β1 integrin activation on all three Ca_L isoforms suggests that this is a fundamental mechanism of Ca_L channel regulation in excitable cells. Extracellular recordings made by other groups in brain slices are largely consistent with our proposal that neuronal Ca^{2+} channels are regulated by ECM-integrin interactions through signaling pathways that include c-Src.[34-36]

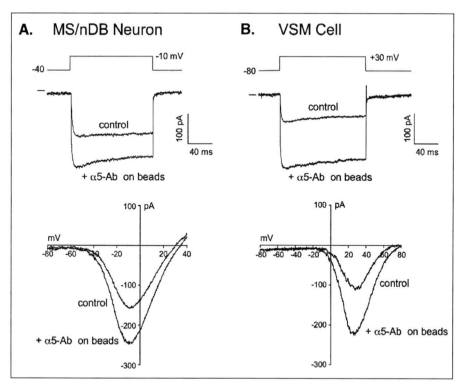

Figure 3. Potentiation of native neuronal and VSM cell Ca_L currents by α5β1 integrin activation. A) whole-cell Ba^{2+} current recordings from a rat MS/nDB (medial septum, diagonal band nucleus) neuron. α5β1 integrin was activated by applying beads coated with anti-α5 integrin Ab from a micropipette positioned close to the cell. The control trace was obtained 2 min after patch rupture; the α5-Ab trace was obtained 4 min after bead application. Current potentiation was 1.6-fold at test potential = −10 mV. N-type and P/Q-type currents were blocked using 5 μM ω-conotoxin MVIIC in the bath at a holding potential (V_H) = −40 mV. The remaining current was blocked >95% by 1 μM nifedipine (not shown). The horizontal line indicates zero current level. The lower panel shows current-voltage relationships obtained from the same cell using a ramp protocol (−100 to +40 mV over 100 ms; V_H = −40 mV). Pipette, 110 mM Cs^+; bath, 2 mM Ba^{2+}. B) whole-cell Ba^{2+} current recordings from a rat arteriolar smooth muscle cell before and after α5β1 integrin activation. Ba^{2+} current potentiation was 2.7-fold 4 min after application of α5-Ab beads. The lower panel shows current-voltage relationship from the same cell obtained using a ramp protocol (V_H = −80 mV). Pipette, 110 mM Cs^+; bath, 20 mM Ba^{2+}. From Gui P. et al. 2006; 281(20):14015-14025;[32] with permission.

Regulation of Ca^{2+}-Dependent Potassium Channels by Integrin Activation

αvβ3 integrin is expressed on both the luminal and abluminal surfaces of the vascular endothelial cells (ECs) and is thought to be involved in several vascular pathologies.[37] It is perhaps not surprising that αvβ3 integrin ligands are capable of acutely regulating vascular tone. For example, RGD peptides (which bind αvβ3, α5β1 and other integrins) have been shown to block flow-induced, EC-dependent vasodilation in coronary arterioles.[9] It has therefore been suggested that soluble αvβ3 integrin ligands may acutely modulate blood flow by interacting with EC integrins.[10,38] Consistent with this observation, EC adhesion to vitronectin, an endogenous αvβ3 integrin ligand, was found to induce an increase in EC $[Ca^{2+}]_i$.[39] Furthermore, acute application

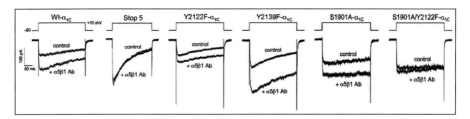

Figure 4. Truncations and single-point mutations identify two critical residues Tyr-2122 (Y2122) and Ser-1901 (S1901). Representative traces showing potentiation of Ba^{2+} current following integrin activation in HEK 293 cells transfected with $β_{1b}$, $α_2δ$ subunits plus WT- $α_{1C-c}$, $α_{1C-c}$ truncation Stop5, single residue α1c-c mutants containing Y2122F, Y2139F or S1901A substitutions, or the double mutant S1901A/Y2122F. Potentiation was not significantly altered in Y2139F, abolished in the Stop5 mutant or the double mutant, but reduced by only ~50% in either the Y2122F mutant or S1901A mutant. Pipette, 110 Cs^+ mM; bath, 20 mM Ba^{2+}. Modified from Gui P. et al. 2006; 281(20):14015-14025;[32] with permission.

of vitronectin or cross-linking of αvβ3 integrin with the LM609 antibody, increased EC $[Ca^{2+}]_i$ and the $[Ca^{2+}]_i$ increase occured as a consequence of tyrosine phosphorylation of phospholipase C-g1 downstream of αvβ3 activation.[39,40]

For these reasons it was proposed that engagement of αvβ3 integrin leads to the activation of an unidentified Ca^{2+} influx pathway.[39] To test this idea, we studied the electrophysiological events underlying αvβ3 integrin-mediated changes in endothelial cell Ca^{2+} signaling using whole-cell patch clamp methods applied to cultured bovine pulmonary artery ECs (the same cells used in ref. 39, 40). The resting membrane potential of the cells averaged -60 ± 3 mV. The application of soluble vitronectin (VN) resulted in activation of an outwardly rectifying K^+ current at potentials from −50 to +50 mV. VN-activated current was significantly inhibited by pretreatment with the αvβ3 integrin antibody LM609, by exchanging extracellular K^+ with Cs^+, or by buffering intracellular Ca^{2+} increases.[41] Collectively, these observations all pointed to a critical role for Ca^{2+}-activated K^+ channels during these events. Indeed, the application of iberiotoxin, a selective inhibitor of large-conductance, Ca^{2+}-activated K^+ (BK) channels, blocked outward current activation in response to VN. Fura-2 microfluorimetry confirmed that VN induced a significant and sustained increase in intracellular Ca^{2+} concentration, although a VN-induced Ca^{2+} current could not be detected.[41]

In light of these findings, we propose that the activation of whole-cell, calcium-activated K^+ current following αvβ3 integrin engagement will hyperpolarize the endothelium, particularly in electrically coupled ECs in vivo,[42] where the resting membrane potential is relatively depolarized. This will sustain the plateau phase of agonist-induced or spontaneous $[Ca^{2+}]_i$ transients by enhancing the electrochemical driving force for Ca^{2+}.[43-45] By this mechanism, αvβ3 engagement by extracellular matrix proteins would be predicted to regulate production of Ca^{2+}-dependent EC vasoactive substances such as endothelium-derived hyperpolarizing factor (EDHF), nitric oxide, prostacyclin and endothelin and thereby acutely modulate vascular tone.[9,10] The idea that Ca^{2+}-activated K^+ channels are regulated by ECM-integrin ligands is consistent with a number of studies on Ca^{2+}-activated K^+ channels and hERG channels in other cell types.[46-48]

Recently, we have found that BK channels in arteriolar smooth muscle cells are also regulated by integrins. In single arteriolar myocytes, activation of α5β1 integrin by an appropriate, insoluble α5β1 antibody resulted in ~30-50% increase in the amplitude of iberiotoxin (IBTX)-sensitive, whole-cell K^+ current.[49] Current potentiation occurred 1-8 min after bead/antibody application to the cell surface. Similarly, FN potentiated IBTX-sensitive K^+ current by up to 80% in some cells. Current potentiation was blocked by the c-Src inhibitor, PP2 (0.1-1 μM). In cell-attached patches, activity of a 230-250 pS K^+ channel, as measured by the product of channel number and open probability ($N·P_o$), was significantly increased after FN application locally to the external surface of cell-attached patches through the recording pipette (Fig. 5). In excised, inside-out patches, FN

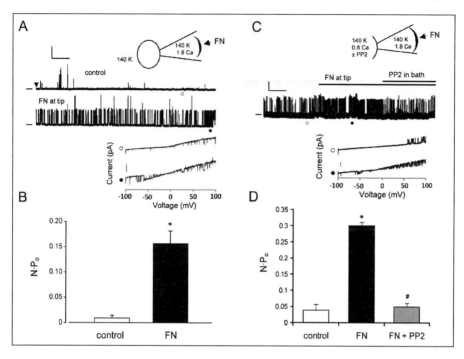

Figure 5. Effect of soluble FN on single channel BK currents in VSM. A) shows data obtained from a cell-attached patch when the pipette was back-filled with FN (15 μg/ml). Top: a diagram of the preparation, illustrating the recording configuration with the cell bathed in 140 mM K+ solution; V_H = +80 mV. The lower inset shows an example of two ramps (−100 to +100 mV) applied during the first minute after seal formation and then after allowing a sufficient amount of time for FN to diffuse to the membrane (respective times are indicated by open and closed symbols). At ~1 min, there were no channel openings at negative potentials but at ~5 min of recording, channel activity was evident at all potentials between −75 and +100 mV. The conductance of the larger amplitude openings was estimated to be 228 pS, which is consistent with a BK channel (representative of 4 cells). B) summary of N·Po values measured from similar protocols before and after FN (n = 4; mean ± SEM). Time controls made in other cells without FN in the pipette showed no significant changes in N·Po over the same time scale. C) current recording from an excised, inside-out patch at +60 mV with solutions as depicted in inset diagram. After FN, PP2 (1 μM) was added to the bath at ~5 min. Calibration bar: 10 pA, 1 min. Inset shows current recordings in response to two voltage ramps (from −100 to +100 mV, 1 sec duration) performed at times indicated by open circle (upper trace) and closed circle (lower trace). Calibration bar for inset: 20 pA. Conductance of the channel in this patch was estimated to be 233 pS from the lower trace. D) summary data for N·P₀ measurements at +80 mV during control, FN and FN+PP2 periods. The average conductance was 242 ± 5 pS for control; 237 ± 4 pS for FN and 238 ± 5 pS for FN+PP2, as estimated from voltage ramps as shown in C. PP3 had no significant effect on N·Po. *, $p < 0.05$ vs control. #, $p < 0.05$ vs FN. Modified from Wu X. et al. 586:1699-1713;[49] with permission.

application through the recording pipette significantly increased N·P₀ and caused a leftward shift in the N·P₀-voltage relationship at constant [Ca^{2+}]. PP2 nearly abolished the effect of FN on channel activity, suggesting that signaling between the integrin and the channel involved a c-Src-mediated increase in Ca^{2+}-sensitivity of the channel via a membrane-delimited pathway.[49]

We have also been able to reproduce this effect in a heterologous expression system. When HEK 293 cells are transfected with the murine BK channel α-subunit (m*Slo*), BK currents can be recorded either in whole-cell mode at low channel density, or in excised macropatches at high channel density.

BK current is consistently potentiated, beginning 1-3 min following α5β1 integrin activation with FN or with α5β1 integrin Ab.[49] Confocal imaging experiments show a substantial degree of colocalization between α5β1 integrin and the BK channel, which is consistent with our observations that excised patches contain all of the protein elements required for channel regulation by integrin activation. The analysis of tail currents recorded in excised macropatches at different calcium concentrations reveals that integrin activation causes a left-shift in the conductance-voltage relation for mSlo at free Ca^{2+} concentrations ≥ 1 µM.[50] In subsequent electrophysiological recordings, we find that overexpression of c-Src with mSlo leads to similar shift in mSlo Ca^{2+} sensitivity, whereas overexpression of catalytically inactive c-Src blocks integrin-induced potentiation.[50] Importantly, neither integrin activation nor c-Src overexpression enhances current if the BK channel contains a point mutation at residue Tyr-766. Thus, BK channel activity in VSM is potentiated by α5β1 integrin activation through an intracellular signaling pathway involving c-Src phosphorylation of the channel α-subunit at Tyr-766. The net result is increased current amplitude, enhanced Ca^{2+} sensitivity and speed of activation of the BK channel, which would collectively promote smooth muscle hyperpolarization in response to α5β1 integrin-FN interactions.[50]

Conclusion: The Physiological Relevance of Coordinated Regulation of Ca_L and BK Channels by Integrins

In VSM, the activation of BK channels promotes vasodilation while the activation of voltage-gated L-type calcium channels promotes vasoconstriction. We have demonstrated that α5β1 integrin signals to both channels, an effect that might seem contradictory. However, careful inspection of the time courses of Ca_L and BK channel potentiation following α5β1 integrin activation reveals that BK channel potentiation is slightly delayed and more sustained.[22,49] Therefore, the net effect of α5β1 integrin activation in VSM is probably to produce a transient increase in Ca^{2+} influx that may subsequently trigger intracellular Ca^{2+} release and other Ca^{2+}-dependent intracellular signaling mechanisms such as PKC activation.

Despite what we have demonstrated in regard to signaling mechanisms between these two ion channels and α5β1 integrins in VSM, many questions remain about the magnitude of the effects in vivo and their physiological role(s). For VSM, it is reasonable to expect that the application of mechanical force, such as that normally associated with an intravascular pressure change, may modify signaling pathways activated by constitutive interactions between FN and α5β1 integrins in the vessel wall. In fact, FN is known to be markedly altered by mechanical stretching, which exposes matricryptic sites that affect cell adhesive signaling as well as self-assembly reactions.[58] We are just beginning to investigate such issues within the vascular wall.

Another more likely example of how ECM-integrin-ion channel interactions impact vascular tone would occur during matrix and/or vessel wall remodeling. Matrix composition of the vessel wall changes as the vessel is remodeled in disease states such as diabetes, hypertension, ischemia-reperfusion injury and atherosclerosis.[51-54] For example, increased deposition of provisional ECM proteins including osteopontin, FN and VN, is observed within the vascular wall during the formation of atherosclerotic plaques. Associated with this and other types of vessel wall remodeling are corresponding changes in both number and type of integrins expressed by VSM and ECs.[55,56] Since it is well documented that such changes in wall protein composition occur in parallel with impaired vascular reactivity,[53,57] a likely contributor to changes in vascular reactivity under these conditions is the signaling between integrins and vascular ion channels.

Finally, another condition in which integrin-ion channel interactions in VSM may be pathologically important occurs whenever there is acute or chronic proteolytic breakdown of the ECM within or surrounding the vessel wall. Proteolytic digestion of the ECM occurs in most inflammatory conditions and in diseases associated with chronic inflammation. For example, proteolytic cleavage of collagen and FN by matrix metalloproteinases (MMPs) results in the production of smaller fragments of those molecules and the exposure of binding sites that are normally cryptic in the native ECM proteins;[58] Type I collagen contains 7 RGD-domains that are normally oriented toward the interior of the triple-helical molecule. When the native protein unfolds following proteolysis, several of these sites become exposed. We have termed fragments of ECM proteins with exposed cryptic sites matricryptins.[58] FN, VN, osteopontin and laminin all contain RGD domains, along with other potential matricryptic sites. Isolated arterioles show no response to native collagen but dilate substantially to proteolytically digested collagen.[12] The dilation is prevented by pretreatment with a β3 integrin blocking antibody,[12] suggesting that it is mediated by the αvβ3 integrin. We propose that αvβ3 may serve a unique role as a matricryptin receptor on VSM and ECs to detect matrix degradation resulting in the production of soluble integrin ligands from proteolytic digestion of normally insoluble ECM proteins. This idea is consistent with our collective observations that VSM Ca_L current is altered only after α5β1 integrin activation by insoluble ligands whereas Ca_L current can be modulated by both insoluble and soluble αvβ3 integrin ligands. Because this is a largely unexplored field of study, it remains to be determined if matricryptins are produced as a result of MMP-mediated digestion of other vascular ECM proteins and if so, if the effects of matricryptins are mediated by modulation of Ca_L and BK channels in vascular cells though their interactions specifically with αvβ3 integrin. A remaining possibility is that other matricryptic receptors exist to work in conjunction with αvβ3 to control these vascular injury responses.

References

1. Vuori K. Integrin signaling: tyrosine phosphorylation events in focal adhesions. J Membr Biol 1998; 165(3):191-9.
2. Larsen M, Artym VV, Green JA et al. The matrix reorganized: extracellular matrix remodeling and integrin signaling. Curr Opin Cell Biol 2006; 18(5):463-71.
3. Schwartz MA. Integrin signaling revisited. Trends Cell Biol 2001; 11:466-470.
4. Giancotti FG, Ruoslahti E. Integrin signaling. Science 1999; 285:1028-1032.
5. Ingber DE. Cellular mechanotransduction: putting all the pieces together. FASEB J 2006; 20(7):811-27.
6. Gao M, Sotomayor M, Villa E et al. Molecular mechanisms of cellular mechanics. Phys Chem Chem Phys 2006; 8(32):3692-706.
7. Glukhova MA, Koteliansky VE. Integrins, cytoskeletal and extracellular matrix proteins in developing smooth muscle cells of human aorta. In: Schwartz SM and Mecham RP, eds. The Vascular Smooth Muscle Cell: Molecular and Biological Responses to the Extracellular Matrix. San Diego, CA: Academic 1995; 37-79.
8. Li YS, Haga JH, Chien S. Molecular basis of the effects of shear stress on vascular endothelial cells. J Biomech 2005; 38(10):1949-71.
9. Muller JM, Chilian WM, Davis MJ. Integrin signaling transduces shear stress-dependent vasodilation of coronary arterioles. Circ Res 1997; 80:320-326.
10. Madden JA, Christman NJ. Integrin signaling, free radicals and tyrosine kinase mediate flow constriction in isolated cerebral arteries. Am J Physiol (Heart Circ Physiol) 1999; 277:H2264-H2271.
11. Mogford JE, Davis GE, Platts SH et al. Vascular smooth muscle αvβ3 integrin mediates arteriolar vasodilation in response to RGD peptides. Circ Res 1996; 79:821-826.
12. Mogford JE, Davis GE, Meininger GA. RGDN peptide interaction with endothelial α5β1 integrin causes sustained endothelin-dependent vasoconstriction of rat skeletal muscle arterioles. J Clin Invest 1997; 100:1647-1653.
13. Lipke DW, Soltis EE, Fiscus RR et al. RGD-containing peptides induce endothelium-dependent and independent vasorelaxations of rat aortic rings. Regul Pept 1996; 63:23-29.
14. Yip KP, Marsh DJ. An Arg-Gly-Asp peptide stimulates constriction in rat afferent arteriole. Am J Physiol (Renal Physiol) 1997; 273:F768-F776.
15. Laplante C, St-Pierre S, Beaulieu AD et al. Small fibronectin fragments induce endothelium-dependent vascular relaxations. Can J Physiol Pharmacol 1988; 66:745-748.
16. Martinez-Lemus LA, Crow T, Davis MJ et al. αvβ3- and α5β1-integrin blockade inhibits myogenic constriction of skeletal muscle resistance arterioles. Am J Physiol (Heart Circ Physiol) 2005; 289:H322-9.
17. Waitkus-Edwards KR, Martinez-Lemus LA, Wu X et al. α4β1Integrin activation of L-type calcium channels in vascular smooth muscle causes arteriole vasoconstriction. Circ Res 2002; 90(4):473-80.
18. Platts, SH, Mogford JE, Davis MJ et al. Role of K+ channels in arteriolar vasodilation mediated by integrin interaction with RGD-containing peptide. Am J Physiol (Heart Circ Physiol) 1998; 275:H1449-H1454.
19. Ledoux J, Werner ME, Brayden JE et al. Calcium-activated potassium channels and the regulation of vascular tone. Physiology 2006; 21:69-78.
20. Davis MJ, Hill MA. Signaling mechanisms underlying the vascular myogenic response. Physiol Rev 1999; 79(2):387-423.

21. D'Angelo G, Mogford JE, Davis GE et al. Integrin-mediated reduction in vascular smooth muscle $[Ca^{2+}]_i$ induced by RGD-containing peptide. Am J Physiol (Heart Circ Physiol) 1999; 272:H2065-H2070.
22. Wu, X, Mogford JE, Platts SH et al. Modulation of calcium current in arteriolar smooth muscle by αvβ3 and α5β1 integrin ligands. J Cell Biol 1998; 143:241-252.
23. Miyamoto S, Akiyama SK, Yamada KM. Synergistic roles for receptor occupancy and aggregation in integrin transmembrane function. Science 1995; 267:883-885.
24. Wu X, Davis GE, Meininger GA et al. Regulation of the L-type calcium channel by α5β1 integrin requires signaling between focal adhesion proteins. J Biol Chem 2001; 276:30285-30292.
25. Wijetunge S, Hughes AD. pp60c-src increases voltage-operated calcium channel currents in vascular smooth muscle cells. Biochem Biophys Res Comm 1995; 217:1039-1044.
26. Wijetunge S, Hughes AD. Activation of endogenous c-Src or a related tyrosine kinase by intracellular (pY)EEI peptide increases voltage-operated calcium channel currents in rabbit ear artery cells. FEBS Lett 1996; 399:63-66.
27. Hu XQ, Singh N, Mukhopadhyay D et al. Modulation of voltage-dependent Ca^{2+} channels in rabbit colonic smooth muscle cells by c-Src and focal adhesion kinase. J Biol Chem 1998; 273:5337-5342.
28. Wijetunge S, Hughes AD. Effect of platelet-derived growth factor on voltage-operated calcium channels in rabbit isolated ear artery cells. Br J Pharmacol 1995; 115:534-538.
29. Gui P, Balasubramanian BB, Wu X et al. Effect of α5β1 integrin activation on heterogenously expressed cardiac L-type calcium channel. Biophysical J 2004; 86(1) 427A.
30. Wang YG, Samarel AM, Lipsius SL. Laminin acts via β1 integrin signalling to alter cholinergic regulation of L-type Ca(2+) current in cat atrial myocytes. J Physiol 2000; 526(1):57-68.
31. Wang YG, Samarel AM, Lipsius SL. Laminin binding to β1-integrins selectively alters beta1- and beta2-adrenoceptor signalling in cat atrial myocytes. J Physiol 2000; 527(1):3-9.
32. Gui P, Wu X, Ling S et al. Integrin receptor activation triggers converging regulation of $Ca_v1.2$ calcium channels by c-Src and protein kinase A pathways. J Biol Chem 2006; 281(20):14015-25.
33. Chao J-T, Gui P, Zamponi G et al. Spatial association between L-type calcium channels and integrins. FASEB J 2007; 21(5):A914.
34. Lin CY, Hilgenberg LG, Smith MA et al. Integrin regulation of cytoplasmic calcium in excitatory neurons depends upon glutamate receptors and release from intracellular stores. Mol Cell Neurosci 2008; 37(4):770-80.
35. Gall CM, Pinkstaff JK, Lauterborn JC et al. Integrins regulate neuronal neurotrophin gene expression through effects on voltage-sensitive calcium channels. Neuroscience 2003; 118(4):925-40.
36. Stäubli U, Chun D, Lynch G. Time-dependent reversal of long-term potentiation by an integrin antagonist. J Neurosci 1998; 18(9):3460-9.
37. Eliceiri BP. Integrin and growth factor receptor crosstalk. Circ Res 2001; 89(12):1104-10.
38. Bryan RM Jr, Marrelli SP, Steenberg ML et al. Effects of luminal shear stress on cerebral arteries and arterioles. Am J Physiol (Heart Circ Physiol) 2001; 280(5):H2011-22.
39. Leavesley DI, Schwartz MA, Rosenfeld M et al. Integrin β1- and β3-mediated endothelial cell migration is triggered through distinct signaling mechanisms. J Cell Biol 1993; 121(1):163-70.
40. Bhattacharya S, Ying X, Fu C et al. αvβ3 integrin induces tyrosine phosphorylation-dependent Ca^{2+} influx in pulmonary endothelial cells. Circ Res 2000; 86(4):456-62.
41. Kawasaki J, Davis GE, Davis MJ. Regulation of Ca^{2+}-dependent K^+ current by αvβ3 integrin engagement in vascular endothelium. J Biol Chem 2004; 279(13):12959-66.
42. Daut J, Mehrke G, Nees S et al. Passive electrical properties and electrogenic sodium transport of cultured guinea-pig coronary endothelial cells. J Physiol 1988; 402:237-54.
43. Peppelenbosch MP, Tertoolen LG, de Laat SW. Epidermal growth factor-activated calcium and potassium channels. J Biol Chem 1991; 266(30):19938-44.
44. Sharma NR, Davis MJ. Mechanism of substance P-induced hyperpolarization of porcine coronary artery endothelial cells. Am J Physiol (Heart Circ Physiol) 1994; 266:H156-64.
45. Vaca L, Licea A, Possani LD. Modulation of cell membrane potential in cultured vascular endothelium. Am J Physiol (Cell Physiol) 1996; 270:C819-24.
46. Hofmann G, Bernabei PA, Crociani O et al. HERG K^+ channels activation during β1 integrin-mediated adhesion to fibronectin induces an up-regulation of αvβ3 integrin in the preosteoclastic leukemia cell line FLG 29.1. J Biol Chem 2001; 276(7):4923-31.
47. Cherubini A, Hofmann G, Pillozzi S et al. Human ether-a-go-go-related gene 1 channels are physically linked to β1 integrins and modulate adhesion-dependent signaling. Mol Biol Cell 2005; 16(6):2972-83.
48. Becchetti A, Arcangeli A, Del Bene MR et al. Response to fibronectin-integrin interaction in leukaemia cells: delayed enhancing of a K^+ current. Proc Biol Sci 1992; 248(1323):235-40.
49. Wu X, Yang Y, Gui P et al. Potentiation of BK channels by α5β1 integrin activation in arteriolar smooth muscle. J Physiol 2008; 586:1699-1713.
50. Yang Y, Wu X, Wu J et al. Integrin activation results in c-Src mediated phosphorylation and potentiation of Maxi K channels. FASEB J 2007; 21(5):A538.

51. Lal H, Guleria RS, Foster DM et al. Integrins: novel therapeutic targets for cardiovascular diseases. Cardiovasc Hematol Agents Med Chem 2007; 5(2):109-32.
52. Hayden MR, Sowers JR, Tyagi SC. The central role of vascular extracellular matrix and basement membrane remodeling in metabolic syndrome and type 2 diabetes: the matrix preloaded. Cardiovasc Diabetol 2005; 4(1):9.
53. del Zoppo GJ, Milner R. Integrin-matrix interactions in the cerebral microvasculature. Arterioscler Thromb Vasc Biol 2006; 26(9):1966-75.
54. Heerkens EH, Izzard AS, Heagerty AM. Integrins, vascular remodeling and hypertension. Hypertension 2007; 49(1):1-4.
55. Scatena M, Liaw L, Giachelli CM. Osteopontin: a multifunctional molecule regulating chronic inflammation and vascular disease. Arterioscler Thromb Vasc Biol 2007; 27(11):2302-9.
56. Intengan HD, Schiffrin EL. Structure and mechanical properties of resistance arteries in hypertension: role of adhesion molecules and extracellular matrix determinants. Hypertension 2000; 36(3):312-8.
57. Hultgårdh-Nilsson A, Durbeej M. Role of the extracellular matrix and its receptors in smooth muscle cell function: implications in vascular development and disease. Curr Opin Lipidol 2007; 18(5):540-5.
58. Davis GE, Bayless KJ, Davis MJ et al. Regulation of tissue injury responses by the exposure of matricryptic sites within extracellular matrix molecules. Am J Pathol 2000; 156:1489-1498.
59. Davis MJ, Wu X, Nurkiewicz T et al. Regulation of ion channels by integrins. Cell Biochemistry and Biophysics 2002; 36(1):41-66.

CHAPTER 8

Adhesion-Dependent Modulation of Macrophage K⁺ Channels

Margaret Colden-Stanfield*

Abstract

Integrin-mediated adhesion of monocytes not only triggers cell rolling and diapedesis, it also activates ionic permeability changes resulting in monocyte activation, maturation and differentiation. Mononuclear phagocytes possess voltage-dependent inwardly rectifying K⁺ (Kir) currents and delayed outwardly, rectifying K⁺ (Kdr) currents that are modulated by tissue origin, adherence, presence of growth factors or cytokines and the functional or differentiation state of the cells. This chapter reviews the exploration of Kir and Kdr channels in mononuclear phagocytes over the last 30 years with an emphasis on culturing conditions, modulation by substrates and role in macrophage function. It has only been recent that successful attempts have been made to study these K⁺ currents in monocytes/macrophages as they may be engaged in the human body which may serve as the foundation for the development of novel therapeutic agents targeting macrophage Kir/Kdr channel activity to favorably influence risk factors for hypertension, atherosclerosis and diabetes.

Introduction

Adhesion of monocytes to extracellular matrix molecules or other cells which is mediated by the engagement of several different families of integrins, not only triggers cell rolling and diapedesis, it also activates other signaling pathways that involve ionic permeability changes resulting in monocyte activation, maturation and differentiation. Mononuclear phagocytes primarily possess three distinct voltage-dependent K⁺ currents: inwardly rectifying (Kir), delayed, outwardly, rectifying (Kdr) as well as inwardly rectifying Ca²⁺-activated K⁺ currents that are modulated by tissue origin, adherence, presence of growth factors or cytokines and the functional or differentiation state of the cells. The characterization of these K⁺ currents has predominantly been performed under in vitro experimental conditions in which immature monocytes or macrophages were attached to nonphysiologic substrates such as tissue culture polystyrene (plastic) or glass coverslips. The characterization of Kir and Kdr currents on polystyrene/glass and their modulation by adherence to more physiologically relevant substrates and their role in monocytic activation/differentiation is the focus of this chapter.

Inwardly Rectifying K⁺ (Kir) Currents

Gallin et al[1-12] have been pioneers in describing K⁺ currents initially in murine spleen macrophages in the mid 70's using high resistance intracellular microelectrode recordings and later in the 80's and 90's with the advent of the patch-clamp technique in macrophages derived from peripheral blood (PB) monocytes isolated by density gradient centrifugation or thioglycollate-induced peritoneal

*Margaret Colden-Stanfield—Morehouse School of Medicine, Department of Physiology, MEB 349, 720 Westview Drive, SW, Atlanta, Georgia 30310, USA.
Email: mstanfield@msm.edu

Integrins and Ion Channels: Molecular Complexes and Signaling, edited by Andrea Becchetti and Annarosa Arcangeli. ©2010 Landes Bioscience and Springer Science+Business Media.

Table 1. Inwardly rectifying K⁺ (Kir) currents in mononuclear phagocytes

Cell Type	Species	Culturing Conditions	Substrate	Characteristics	Blockers	Ref
THP-1 monocytes	Human	5 h to 3 days	Glass/Poly	~8% of cells	Ba^{2+}, Cs	30-34
U937 monocytes	Human	30 min to 4 h	Poly	48% of cells, 51 pS, PMA-diff. monocyte-like		15
PB macrophages	Human	30 min to 4 h	Poly	37 pS	Cs	15
PB macrophages	Human	5 days or more	Glass	33% of cells, 28 pS, V$_{rest}$ −56 mV	Ba^{2+}, Cs	9, 11
PB macrophages	Human	up to 3 wks	Poly	V$_{rest}$ −34 mV	Ba^{2+}	13-14
HL-60 macrophages	Human	4-6 days PMA-diff	Glass	IP$_3$, IP$_4$	Ba^{2+}, Cs, CSF-1, GTPγS, RA-diff.	29
THP-1 macrophages	Human	3 days PMA-diff	Glass	70% of cells, 30 pS, Kir2.1	Ba^{2+}, Cs	30-31
THP-1 macrophages	Human	5 h	LPS-ECs, VCAM-1 α-VLA-4x	74% of cells, Kir2.1, V$_{rest}$ −40 mV, V$_{rest}$ ≥ −55 mV Kir alone, ⇑ Ca^{2+} entry, ⇑ IL-8 Production	Ba^{2+}, Cs	32-34
Spleen macrophages	Murine				Ba^{2+}	5
Peritoneal Macrophages	Murine	Day 5 to 2 wks	Glass	35% of cells, V$_{rest}$ −80 mV, washout, internal GDPβS or ATP	Ba^{2+}, Cs$^+$, Rb$^+$	3-4, 17, 21
J774.1 macrophages	Murine	<24 h	Glass	V$_{rest}$ −58mV, 29 pS, washout Leishmania amazonensis infection	Ba^{2+}, LPS, GTPγS	17, 22
J774.1 macrophages	Murine	>1 day	Poly	V$_{rest}$ −78 mV, Kir2.1	GTPγS	16, 19-20
Brain macrophages	Murine	1-3 days	Glass	ameboid	GTPγS	41

continued on next page

Table 1. Continued

Cell Type	Species	Culturing Conditions	Substrate	Characteristics	Blockers	Ref
BM macrophages	Murine	7 days M-CSF (10%L929CM)	Poly	94% of cells, Kir2.1, M-CSF	Ba^{2+}, Cs^+, LPS, TNFα	36
Brain macrophages	Murine	10 days M-CSF (30%L929CM)	Glass	97% of cells, V_{rest} of −66 mV		42
BM macrophages	Murine	7 days M-CSF (20%L929CM)	α-VLA-4x	V_{rest} −46 mV, Kir2.1	↓α-VLA-4x, Cs	
Peritoneal macrophages	Rat	5 h	Poly	⇑ longer incubation		37-38
Brain macrophages	Rat	2 h to 5 days	Poly, Poly-L-lysine Glass	V_{rest} −67 mV, 30 pS, LPS, washout ameboid	TEA, 4-AP, Ba^{2+} Cs^+	37-38, 40, 56-57

Abbreviations: Poly: polystyrene; PMA-diff: 3-day phorbol 12-myristate 13-acetate-differentiated; PB: peripheral blood; V_{rest}: resting membrane potential; CSF-1: colony-stimulating factor-1; RA-diff: retinoic acid-differentiated; LPS-ECS: 24-h lipopolysaccharide-treated human umbilical vein endothelial cells; VCAM-1: vascular cell adhesion molecule-1; αVLA-4x: crosslinked mAbVLA-4; IL-8: interleukin-8; M-CSF: macrophage colony-stimulating factor; TNFα: tumor necrosis factor-α.

macrophages. Table 1 summarizes the salient features of Kir currents in monocyte/macrophages. Kir currents are present in 33% of long-term cultured human PB-derived macrophages and are characterized by (1) activation at potentials negative to −60 mV, (2) better conduction of inward current than outward current, (3) dependence on voltage and extracellular K⁺ concentration, (4) inactivation at more negative potentials, (5) block by Ba^{2+}, Cs^+ and Rb^+, (6) Kir2.1 subunit primarily underlying the functional current and (7) the ability to set resting membrane potential (V_{rest}) closer to E_K.[9,11,13-14] As 28 pS Kir channels are believed to underlie the macroscopic whole-cell Kir currents in human macrophages adherent to uncoated glass, a similar 37 pS Kir channel is evident in PB-derived macrophages adherent to uncoated polystyrene for less than 4 h.[15] Murine J774.1 macrophages (29 pS) and peritoneal macrophages adherent to polystyrene or glass for periods of 1 to 14 days possess larger amplitude Kir currents than acutely adherent cells.[3-4,16-22] The current decays over time once the whole-cell configuration is established (washout). G protein activators such as GTPγS enhance the rate of washout while preventing the activation of G proteins with GDPβS stabilizes whole-cell Kir currents.[18-21] Overnight exposure to exogenous negative bacterial endotoxin, lipopolysaccharide (LPS), reduces Kir magnitude in J774.1 macrophages.[19] Although acutely applied (5 min) exogenous LPS does not affect Kir currents, a 60-90 min exposure to intracellular LPS completely attenuates Kir currents in human macrophages.[23] The ability to express and functionally record J774.1 Kir currents in Xenopus oocytes and subsequent isolation and cloning of cDNA encoding for IRK1 Kir channels from J774.1 macrophages provided the original classification of Kir channels in macrophages at the molecular level.[24-25]

The use of immortalized human tumor cell lines such as U-937, HL-60 and THP-1 cells has afforded additional strategies to further describe Kir and Kdr currents and their possible involvement in monocyte differentiation.[26-28] While all three cancer cell lines can be differentiated with phorbol esters, Vitamin D_3 and/or TGF-β to mature macrophages, the HL-60 cell line can also be directed to a neutrophil lineage with exposure to retinoic acid or dimethyl sulfoxide. U-937 monocytes exposed to phorbol 12-myristate 13-acetate (PMA) display 51 pS Kir channels in 48% of the cells.[15] Similarly, Kir currents predominate in HL-60 cells differentiated to macrophages by 4-6 days of PMA treatment and can be attenuated by exposure to colony stimulating factor-1 (CSF-1) and GTPγS.[29] THP-1 monocytes exhibit many of the K⁺ conductances present in primary monocytes and macrophages and when present set V_{rest} to more negative levels.[30-31] That is, a small percentage of cells possess Kir currents in immature THP-1 monocytes even after 3 days of adherence to glass or polystyrene. When differentiated to macrophages by PMA treatment, the majority of THP-1 macrophages possess 30 pS Kir channels that underlie the Ba^{2+}- and Cs^+-sensitive Kir currents. IRK1 mRNA expression, also known as Kir2.1, is significantly enhanced in PMA-differentiated THP-1 macrophages.[30-31]

Since THP-1 cells display a variety of adhesion molecules on their surface that mediate their interactions with extracellular matrix molecules and other cells, much of our work has been performed in this monocytic cell line to examine the effects of integrin-ligand interactions on the membrane conductances in monocytes. Our initial novel reporting that a similar Kir current is induced by adherence of THP-1 monocytes to activated endothelial cells (ECs) or purified VCAM-1 suggests that the presence of the Kir current may be involved in monocyte activation and/or differentiation (Fig. 1).[32] We found that when THP-1 cells are bound to uncoated polystyrene (plastic) or unstimulated EC monolayers for 1-5 h only a small percentage of cells (6-14%) possessed Kir currents with a depolarized V_{rest} (−19 to −24 mV) (Fig. 1B and D). However, when THP-1 cells become adherent to 24-h lipopolysaccharide (LPS)-treated EC monolayers or purified VCAM-1, Kir currents are expressed in 73-81% of the cells which hyperpolarizes the cells by about 20 mV (Fig. 1A and C). Even a brief (15 min) interaction between THP-1 cells and activated endothelial cell monolayers is sufficient to trigger early signaling events such as the initiation of de novo protein synthesis and tyrosine phosphorylation to induce Kir currents 5 h later. It is the specific interaction of upregulated endothelial or purified VCAM-1 with integrin ligand, very late antigen-4 (VLA-4, α4β1), on the surface of THP-1 monocytes that triggers VLA-4 integrin clustering (Fig. 2) and the time-dependent induction of Kir currents.[33] Immunocytochemical stain-

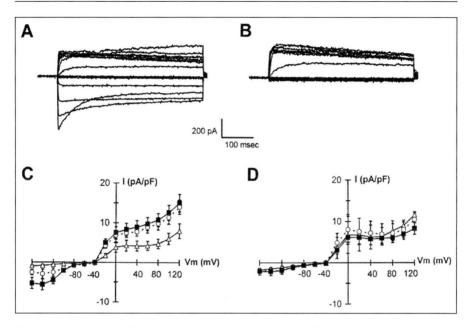

Figure 1. A family of digitized whole-cell currents recorded in THP-1 monocytes adherent to (A) 24-h LPS-activated umbilical vein endothelial cells (LPS-ECs) or (B) polystyrene for 5 h. A 450-msec pulse stepping from −160 mV to +120 mV in 20-mV increments was delivered every 1 sec from a holding potential of −40 mV. Current density-voltage relationships obtained from THP-1 monocytes adherent to (C) LPS-ECs or (D) polystyrene for 1 (Δ), 3 (O), or 5 h (■). Current amplitude for all current density-voltage relations was measured during the last 50 msec of each voltage step and then normalized to C_m. Each plotted point is the mean ± SEM of current densitiestaken from 5-18 cells. (Adapted from Colden-Stanfield and Gallin, 1998,[32] used with permission of The American Physiological Society.)

ing provides direct evidence that VLA-4 integrin clustering occurs on the surface of THP-1 cells when cells are adherent to LPS-ECs or immobilized VCAM-1. The engagement and clustering of VLA-4 integrins produces a Cs^+-sensitive hyperpolarization of V_{rest} that augments store-depleted Ca^{2+} influx to enhance Ca^{2+}-mediated interleukin-8 (IL-8) production (Fig. 3), all of which can be mimicked by THP-1 cell interaction with crosslinked, immobilized antibody raised against VLA-4 (αVLA-4x).[32-34] Preliminary real-time RT-PCR analyses in our laboratory revealed a 3-fold increase in Kir2.1 (IRK1) mRNA in THP-1 cells with clustered VLA-4 integrins compared to THP-1 monocytes bound to polystyrene. We observed a similar augmentation in Kir2.1 mRNA levels in PMA-differentiated THP-1 macrophages compared to undifferentiated THP-1 monocytes (unpublished observations).

Eder and Fischer[35] first described the presence of Kir channels in the majority of murine bone marrow-derived macrophages (BMDMs) cultured for 7 days on polystyrene in the presence of medium supplemented with supernatant of L-929 fibroblast conditioned media (30%L-929CM) as a source of macrophage colony-stimulating factor (M-CSF). Subsequently, Vicente et al[36] more fully characterized analogous Ba^{2+}- or Cs^+- sensitive Kir currents by demonstrating the presence of Kir2.1 mRNA and protein levels in murine BMDMs cultured under identical culturing conditions which may regulate proliferation processes in these cells. Interestingly, extended treatment with exogenous LPS or TNFα significantly reduced Kir2.1 mRNA and protein levels and the magnitude of Kir currents in these cells. More recently, we have extended our research focus to murine BMDMs in our efforts to better understand the role of K^+ transport mechanisms in events leading to macrophage activation/differentiation and cardiovascular disease states such as hypertension and

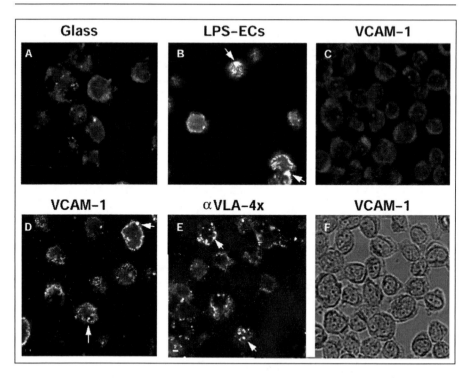

Figure 2. Immunocytochemical staining of VLA-4 surface antigen on THP-1 monocytes adherent to (A) glass (B) lipopolysaccharide-treated HUVECs (LPS-ECs), (D) immobilized VCAM-1 or (E) crosslinked mAbVLA-4 (αVLA-4x) for 5 h. Arrows indicate clustering of VLA-4 integrins. (C) Low nonspecific staining on THP-1 monocytes adherent to VCAM-1 in the presence of secondary antibody alone with corresponding transmitted light image (F). Bar in (E) denotes 2 μm for all images. (Adapted from Colden-Stanfield, 2002,[33] used with permission of The American Physiological Society.)

atherosclerosis. Our initial experiments in murine BMDMs that were first cultured in suspension in Teflon jars for 7 to 11 days with 20%L-929CM-supplemented medium and then attached to polystyrene for <1 h revealed the exclusive presence of Cs^+-sensitive Kir currents that increased in magnitude about 3-fold from Day 7 to Day 11 and correlated well with Kir2.1 mRNA expression levels (Fig. 4A and C, unpublished observations). A lack of Kdr currents in these cells is not in agreement with previous reports in murine BMDMs[35-36] and may be explained by the different culturing conditions of 20%L-929CM and suspension cultures. Our preliminary experiments performed in murine BMDMs with clustered VLA-4 integrins revealed an increased expression of Kdr currents accompanied by reduced Kir currents (Fig. 4A-C). Blockade of VLA-4-induced Kdr currents by margatoxin suggest that Kv1.3 underlies the VLA-4-induced Kdr current elicited during depolarization (Fig. 4D).

A growing body of work studying ion transport mechanisms in brain microglial cells, the resident macrophages of the central nervous system, confirms the predominant presence of similar Kir currents with 30 pS single-channel conductance in cells cultured on polystyrene up to 2 weeks that possess an ameboid shape reflective of a mature macrophage-like morphology.[37-41] A parallel phenomenon occurs in brain macrophages in that culturing microglial cells with M-CSF enhances the magnitude of Kir currents.[42-43] mRNA expression of two of the four Kir subfamilies, IRK1 and ROMK1, have been described in brain macrophages while

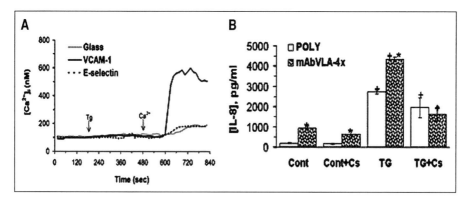

Figure 3. A) Changes in [Ca^{2+}]$_i$ in THP-1 monocytes adherent to various substrates. Representative tracings of [Ca^{2+}]$_i$ changes that occur in individual THP-1 monocytes adherent to glass, immobilized VCAM-1 or E-selectin for 5 h after the addition of thapsigargin, (Tg 100 nM), a Ca^{2+}-ATPase inhibitor and CaCl$_2$ (1 mM). Fura-2-loaded cells were incubated in Ca^{2+}-free saline solution before addition of Tg to deplete Ca^{2+} stores to trigger Ca^{2+} entry after readditon of external CaCl$_2$. (Adapted from Colden-Stanfield and Scanlon, 2000,[34] used with permission of The American Physiological Society.) B) Basal (Cont) and stimulated IL-8 (thapsigargin, TG) release from THP-1 monocytes adherent to POLY or mAbVLA4x for 5 h in the absence or presence of CsCl (10 mM). Each bar is the mean ± SE of supernatant IL-8 of 3 independent experiments performed in duplicate. *Significantly different from the corresponding POLY group. +Significantly different the control group. (Adapted from Colden-Stanfield, 2002,[33] used with permission of The American Physiological Society.)

G proteins and LPS activation modulate these currents implicating a role of the GIRK Kir subfamily.[44-45]

Physiologic and Pathophysiologic Roles of Macrophage Kir Channels

Kir channels play pivotal roles in maintenance of V$_{rest}$, regulation of the action potential duration, receptor-dependent inhibition of cellular excitability, secretion and absorption of K$^+$ ions across cell membranes and differentiation of several cell types including monocytes, mast cells, cardiomyocytes, skeletal muscle and neuroblastoma cells.[46-49] Monocytes are among the first cells present in lesion-prone areas in the development and progression of atherosclerosis. Upon exposure to a variety of signals, monocytes rapidly differentiate into tissue macrophages in the vascular intima. Our work with VLA-4 integrin clustering in THP-1 monocytes/macrophages provides evidence to suggest that long-lived macrophages accumulated at sites of chronic inflammation associated with cardiometabolic disease states are likely to have greater expression of Kir currents which may act as an early signaling event in monocyte differentiation. Mature macrophages express multiple scavenger receptors that facilitate internalization of modified lipoproteins, leading to the development of cholesterol-laden foam cells.[50] Lei et al[51-53] recently postulated that the expression of Kir and Kdr currents may modulate human monocyte-derived macrophage differentiation into foam cells. Uptake of oxidized low density lipoprotein (oxLDL) into human PB-derived macrophages over a 60 h-period is accompanied by increased cellular total cholesterol, free cholesterol and cholesterol ester. Even though Kir2.1 and Kv1.3 mRNA and protein levels are unchanged during foam cell formation, exposure to BaCl$_2$ (Kir2.1 blocker) or margatoxin (Kv1.3 blocker) reduces cellular cholesterol content following uptake of oxLDL, observations that merit further examination.

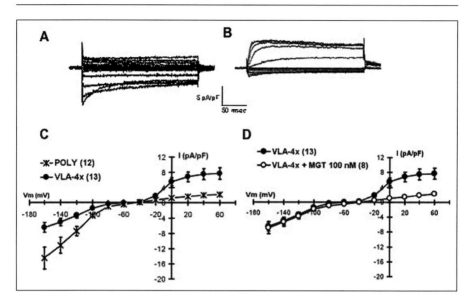

Figure 4. A family of digitized whole-cell currents recorded in BM-derived macrophages adherent to (A) polystyrene (POLY) or (B) immobilized, crosslinked anti-VLA-4 (VLA-4x) for 5 h. A 250-msec pulse stepping from −160 mV to +60 mV in 20-mV increments was delivered every 1 sec from a holding potential of −40 mV. Current density-voltage relationships obtained from BM-derived macrophages adherent to (C) POLY (∗) or VLA-4x (•) for 5 h and (D) with clustered VLA-4 integrins in the absence (•) or presence of the selective Kv1.3 blocker, margatoxin (O). Current amplitude for all current density-voltage relations was measured during the first 50 msec of each voltage step and then normalized to C_m. Each plotted point is the mean ± SEM of current densities taken from 8-13 cells. (Unpublished observations).

Delayed, Outwardly Rectifying K⁺ (Kdr) Currents

Delayed, outwardly rectifying K⁺ (Kdr) currents in monocytes/macrophages are typically characterized by 1) a threshold activation voltage at approximately −40 mV, 2) inhibition by charybdotoxin, tetraethylammonium chloride, 4-aminopyridine and margatoxin, 3) contributing to a more depolarized V_{rest}, 4) inactivation at potentials positive to +30 mV and 5) Kv1.3 subunit primarily underlying the functional current. Kdr currents are expressed in the majority of rat and murine peritoneal macrophages,[54] murine J774.1 macrophages,[16] human monocytes/macrophages[23,31-34] and brain macrophages[41,55-56] adherent to polystyrene or glass for 1-4 days (Table 2). A less robust Kdr expression is evident in longer-term cultures at a time when Kir currents predominate (Table 1) suggesting a reduction of Kdr current as these cells develop into mature macrophages.[17] Conversely, 50% of alveolar macrophages express 4-AP-sensitive Kdr currents after the cells have been bound to polystyrene for a week.[13] Human PB monocytes incubated on a confluent astrocyte monolayer for 2 weeks possess Kir currents but newly express Kdr currents.[57] Our work with THP-1 monocytes has revealed that although most cells (75%) express Kdr currents regardless of substrate, the magnitude of the Kdr currents is significantly reduced when the cells are adherent to unstimulated ECs, purified E-selectin, VCAM-1 and αVLA-4x compared to polystyrene or LPS-ECs, an observation that warrants further investigation.[32-34] Interestingly, our initial recordings in murine BM-derived macrophages illustrates enhanced expression and amplitude levels of Kdr currents when VLA-4 integrins were clustered with αVLA-4x (Fig. 4).

A yin-yang relationship between Kir and Kdr expression levels in monocytes/macrophages is supported by our observations in human THP-1 cells in that there appears to be a balance of expression of these channels as it relates to substrates.[32-34] Cells that predominantly express Kir over Kdr currents are more hyperpolarized approaching E_K. Blockade of Kdr currents in cells possessing both types of K+ channels become more hyperpolarized indicating that the relative presence of each current contributes to V_{rest}. Treatment of murine BM with granulocyte macrophage colony-stimulating factor (GM-CSF) for 7 days to produce neutrophils and immature monocytes predominantly express Kdr currents while treatment of BM with macrophage colony-stimulating factor (M-CSF) to generate mature macrophages largely express Kir currents.[35-36] Furthermore, in a protocol which promotes macrophage proliferation, the response to LPS or TNFα is stimulatory for Kdr currents but inhibitory for Kir currents in BM-derived macrophages. A preliminary study of K+ currents in BM-derived macrophages under our culturing and recording conditions demonstrated the absence of Kdr currents until cells were incubated on αVLA-4x for 5 h (Fig. 4) which was paralleled by Kv1.3 mRNA levels. A similar yin-yang phenomenon occurs with Kir and Kdr currents when brain microglial cells are treated for 10 days with M-CSF to produce macrophages or granulocyte macrophage colony-stimulating factor (GM-CSF) to produce neutrophils and immature monocytes.[42] M-CSF–treated microglia have a V_{rest} of −66 mV with 75% of cells possessing Kir currents alone and less than 1% only expressing Kdr currents. In contrast, GM-CSF-treated microglia have a V_{rest} of −59 mV, 48% of cells only express Kdr currents and 12% of cells only possess Kir currents. Further incubation of M-CSF-treated microglia with GM-CSF pushes the cells to express more Kdr currents. Predominant Kir channel expression may be a prerequisite early signaling event for macrophage differentiation as predominant Kdr channel expression may be for macrophage activation.

Physiologic and Pathophysiologic Roles of Macrophage Kdr Channels

Efforts studying the functional role of Kdr currents in macrophages have focused on their involvement in activation processes and the ability to proliferate. Using a protocol that inhibits proliferation but activates cells, Vicente et al[36] demonstrated that G_o-arrested BM-derived macrophages treated with LPS or TNF for 24 hrs significantly increases Kdr mRNA and protein levels which underlies enhanced functional whole-cell currents. Single-channel recordings illustrate that Fc-mediated phagocytosis of latex beads by human PB-derived macrophages incubated on glass 1-3 weeks is associated with enhanced inward and outward K+ currents.[58] On the other hand, phagocytosis of zymosan, a pathogen extract from *Saccharomyces cerevisiae*, is not affected by microinjected LPS, which reduces both whole-cell Kir and Kdr currents in human PB-derived macrophages adherent to polystyrene for 1 week.[23] The capacity of brain microglial cells to act as antigen presenting cells is optimal when microglial are treated with GM-CSF, a setting in which Kdr currents predominate.[42] LPS activation of rat brain microglial cells also induces Kv1.3 and Kv1.6 mRNA expression within 2-3 h of LPS exposure.[44] In murine microglial cells both Kv1.3 and Kv1.5 channel subunit expression is required for the LPS-induced Kdr current and by employing a Kv1.5−/− knockout mouse and an antisense approach, Pannasch et al[59] showed that LPS-induced nitric oxide release from murine microglia is reduced in the absence of Kv1.5 in microglia. Margatoxin treatment has also been shown to reduce migration of rat brain macrophages on a fibronectin matrix implicating a role of Kv1.3 channel in this integrin-dependent macrophage function.[60]

M-CSF dependent proliferation is inhibited by margatoxin and is accompanied by augmented Kv1.3 expression levels confirming a role of Kv1.3 in BM-derived macrophage proliferation.[36] LPS- or TNF-stimulated iNOS protein expression was also inhibited by margatoxin indicating a role of Kv1.3 in macrophage activation. Vicente et al[61] further characterized in BM-derived macrophages the expression of Kvβ subunit, their modulation by proliferation and the mode of activation and impact on Kdr current inactivation kinetics. More recently, the co-assembly of Kv1.5 and Kv1.3 subunits to form heterotetrameric channels in BM-derived macrophages influences Kdr current kinetics and could possibly affect macrophage function and potential therapeutic strategies in treating autoimmune and cardiometabolic diseases.[62-64]

Table 2. Delayed, outwardly rectifying K⁺ (Kdr) currents in mononuclear phagocytes

Cell Type	Species	Culturing Conditions	Substrate	Characteristics	Blockers	Ref
THP-1 monocytes	Human	5 h	Poly Basal ECs E-selectin	~72% of cells, V_{rest} −22 mV	ChTx, TEA, 4-AP	32-34
THP-1 monocytes	Human	3 days	Glass	99% of cells, Kv1.3	TEA, PMA-diff.	30-31
PB macrophages	Human	5 days or more	Glass	LPS	Cs⁺	23
PB macrophages	Human	1-3 wks	Glass	Fc-mediated phagocytosis, LPS, 35 pS		58
THP-1 macrophages	Human	5 h	LPS-ECs VCAM-1 αVLA-4x	~79% of cells, Kv1.3, V_{rest} −40 mV	ChTx, TEA	32-34
Alveolar macrophages	Human	1 wk	Poly	50% of cells	4-AP	13-14
Peritoneal macrophages	Murine	1-2 days	Poly	⇑ by flow	⇓ by 5-6 days in culture	17
Peritoneal macrophages	Murine	1-4 days	Poly	96% of cells, V_{rest} −85 mV, 16 pS	4-AP	54
Peritoneal macrophages	Murine	Up to 2 wks	Poly	IP₃		21
J774.1 macrophages	Murine	<24 h	Poly	GTPγS, washout	4-AP	16
J774.1 macrophages	Murine	1-2 days	Poly	⇑ by flow	⇓ by 5-6 days in culture	17

continued on next page

Table 2. Continued

Cell Type	Species	Culturing Conditions	Substrate	Characteristics	Blockers	Ref
Brain macrophages	Murine	1-3 days	Glass			41
Brain monocytes/PMNs	Murine	10 days GM-CSF	Glass	74% of cells, V_{rest} −59 mV		42
BM monocytes/PMNs	Murine	7 days GM-CSF	Poly	97% of cells LPS, TNFα		35-36
BM macrophages	Murine	7 days M-CSF (30%L929CM)	Poly	Kv1.3, Kv1.5, Kvβ subunits Kv1.3 modulated by Kv1.5, LPS, TNF	MgTx	36, 61-63
BM macrophages	Murine	7 days M-CSF (20%L929CM)	α-VLA-4x	Kv1.3	MgTx	
Peritoneal macrophages	Rat	5 h	Poly	LPS, washout		13-14
Brain macrophages	Rat	1-24 h	Poly, Glass		4-AP, TEA, ChTX	37-38, 40, 56-57

Abbreviations: Basal ECs: unstimulated endothelial cells; ChTX: charybdotoxin; TEA: tetraethylammonium chloride; 4-AP: 4-aminopyridine; MgTx; Margatoxin. Refer to Table 1 for explanation of all other abbreviations.

Conclusion

This chapter reviewed the exploration of Kir and Kdr channels in mononuclear phagocytes over the last 30 years with an emphasis on culturing conditions, modulation by substrates and role in macrophage function. It has only been recent that successful attempts have been made to study these K^+ currents in monocytes/macrophages as they may be engaged in the human body. Further studies will be necessary to determine the expression levels of other members of the Kir subfamilies: GIRK, ROMK1 and ATPK. As we have demonstrated with chemokine production,[33] respiratory burst and other functional endpoints for macrophages are most likely to be enhanced when Kir currents predominate. With the recent introduction of silencing genes through RNA interference technology[65-66] and the eventual development of more selective K^+ blockers, the identity and role of Kir and Kdr channels in macrophage chemotaxis, the ability to produce a respiratory burst, generate cytokines, engulf pathogens and become a foam cell will most assuredly be elucidated. The study of macrophages isolated from a recently developed mouse with a point mutation ($\alpha 4Y991A$) that blocks $\alpha 4$ integrin signaling[67] and possesses reduced metabolic consequences of high fat diet-induced obesity provides an alternative approach to determining the link between integrin-mediated K^+ channel activity and macrophage function. These new insights can then be applied in the development of therapeutic agents targeting macrophage Kir/Kdr channel activity to favorably influence risk factors for hypertension, atherosclerosis and diabetes.

Acknowledgments

I would like to thank Drs. Pamela Gunter-Smith and Gary Gibbons for providing feedback on this chapter.

References

1. Gallin EK, Wiederhold M, Lipskey P et al. Spontaneous and induced membrane hyperpolarization in macrophages. J Cell Physol 1975; 86:653-662.
2. Gallin EK, Gallin JJ. Interaction of chemotactic factors with human macrophages. Induction of transmembrane potential changes. J Cell Physol 1977; 75:160-166.
3. Gallin EK, Livengood DR. Nonlinear current-voltage relationships in cultured macrophages. J Cell Biol 1980; 85(1):160-165.
4. Gallin EK, Livengood DR. Inward rectification in mouse macrophages: evidence for a negative resistance region. Am J Physiol 1981; 241(1):C9-C17.
5. Gallin EK. Voltage clamp studies in macrophages from mouse spleen cultures. Science 1981; 214(4519):458-460.
6. Gallin EK. Electrophysiological properties of macrophages. Fed Proc 1984; 43(9):2385-2389.
7. Gallin EK. Calcium- and voltage-activated potassium channels in human macrophages. Biophys J 1984; 46(6):821-825.
8. Gallin EK. Ionic channels in leukocytes. J Leukoc Biol 1986; 39(3):241-254.
9. Gallin EK. Evidence for Ca-activated inwardly rectifying K^+ channels in human macrophages. Am J Physiol 1989; 257(1 Pt 1):C77-C85.
10. Gallin EK. Ion channels in leukocytes. Physiol Rev 1991; 71(3):775-811.
11. Gallin EK, McKinney LC. Patch-clamp studies in human macrophages: single-channel and whole-cell characterization of two K^+ conductances. J Membr Biol 1988; 103(1):55-66.
12. Gallin EK, Grinstein S. Ion channels and carriers in leukocytes: distribution and functional role. In: Gallin JI, Goldstein IM and R. Snyderman, eds. Inflammation: Basic Principles and Clinical Correlates, Second Edition; New York: Raven Press, Ltd, 1992:441-458.
13. Nelson DJ, Jow B, Popovich KJ. Whole-cell currents in macrophages: II. Alveolar macrophages. J Membr Biol 1990; 117(1):45-55.
14. Nelson DJ, Jow B, Jow F. Lipopolysaccharide induction of outward potassium current expression in human monocyte-derived macrophages: lack of correlation with secretion. J Membr Biol 1992; 125(3):207-218.
15. McCann FV, Keller TM, Guyre PM. Ion channels in human macrophages compared with the U-937 cell line. J Membr Biol 1987; 96(1):57-64.
16. Gallin EK, Sheehy PA. Differential expression of inward and outward potassium currents in the macrophage-like cell line J774.1. J Physiol 1985; 369:475-499.
17. Randriamampita C, Trautmann A. Ionic channels in murine macrophages. J Cell Biol 1987; 105(2):761-769.

18. McKinney LC, Gallin EK. Inwardly rectifying whole-cell and single-channel K⁺ currents in the murine macrophage cell line J774.1. J Membr Biol 1988; 103(1):41-53.
19. McKinney LC, Gallin EK. Effect of adherence, cell morphology and lipopolysaccharide on potassium conductance and passive membrane properties of murine macrophage J774.1 cells. J Membr Biol 1990; 116(1):47-56.
20. McKinney LC, Gallin EK. G-protein activators induce a potassium conductance in murine macrophages. J Membr Biol 1992; 130(3):265-276.
21. Judge SI, Montcalm-Mazzilli E, Gallin EK. I$_{Kir}$ regulation in murine macrophages: whole cell and perforated patch studies. Am J Physiol 1994; 267(6 Pt 1):C1691-C1698.
22. Forero ME, Marín M, Corrales Am et al. Leishmania amazonensis infection induces changes in the electrophysiological properties of macrophage-like cells. J Membr Biol 1999; 170(2):173-180.
23. Gerth A, Grosche J, Nieber K et al. Intracellular LPS inhibits the activity of potassium channels and fails to activate NFkappaB in human macrophages. J Cell Physiol 2005; 202(2):442-452.
24. Perier F, Coulter KL, Radeke CM et al. Expression of an inwardly rectifying potassium channel in xenopus oocytes. J Neurochem 1992; 59:1971-1974.
25. Kubo Y, Baldwin TJ, Jan YN et al. Primary structure and functional expression of a mouse inward rectifier potassium channel. Nature 1993; 362(6416):127-133.
26. Sundström C, Nilsson K. Establishment and characterization of a human histiocytic lymphoma cell line (U-937). Int J Cancer 1976; 17(5):565-577.
27. Collins SJ, Ruscetti FW, Gallagher RE et al. Terminal differentiation of human promyelocytic leukemia cells induced by dimethyl sulfoxide and other polar compounds. Proc Natl Acad Sci USA 1978; 75(5):2458-2462.
28. Auwerx, J. The human leukemia cell line, THP-1: A multifacetted model for the study of monocyte-macrophage differentiation. Experientia 1991; 47:22-31.
29. Wieland SJ, Chou RH, Gong QH. Macrophage-colony-stimulating factor (CSF-1) modulates a differentiation-specific inward-rectifying potassium current in human leukemic (HL-60) cells. J Cell Physiol 1990; 142(3):643-651.
30. Kim SY, Silver MR, DeCoursey TE. Ion channels in human THP-1 monocytes. J Membr Biol 1996; 152(2):117-130.
31. DeCoursey TE, Kim SY, Silver MR et al. Ion channel expression in PMA-differentiated human THP-1 macrophages. J Membr Biol 1996; 152(2):141-157.
32. Colden-Stanfield M, Gallin EK. Modulation of K⁺ currents in monocytes by VCAM-1 and E-selectin on activated human endothelium. Am J Physiol Cell Physiol 1998; 275(1 Pt 1):C267-C277.
33. Colden-Stanfield M. Clustering of very late antigen-4 integrins modulates K⁺ currents to alter Ca^{2+}-mediated monocyte function. Am J Physiol Cell Physiol 2002; 283(3):C990-C1000.
34. Colden-Stanfield M, Scanlon M. VCAM-1-induced inwardly rectifying K⁺ current enhances Ca^{2+} entry in human THP-1 monocytes. Am J Physiol Cell Physiol 2000; 279(2):C488-C494.
35. Eder C, Fischer HG. Effects of colony-stimulating factors on voltage-gated K⁺ currents of bone marrow-derived macrophages. Naunyn Schmiedebergs Arch Pharmacol 1997; 355(2):198-202.
36. Vicente R, Escalada A, Coma M et al. Differential voltage-dependent K⁺ channel responses during proliferation and activation in macrophages. J Biol Chem 2003; 278(47):46307-46320. Epub 2003. Erratum in: J Biol Chem 2005; 280(13):13204.
37. Kettenmann H, Hoppe D, Gottmann K et al. Cultured microglial cells have a distinct pattern of membrane channels different from peritoneal macrophages. J Neurosci Res 1990; 26(3):278-287.
38. Kettenmann H, Banati R, Walz W. Electrophysiological behavior of microglia. Glia 1993; 7(1):93-101.
39. Korotzer AR, Cotman CW. Voltage-gated currents expressed by rat microglia in culture. Glia 1992; 6(2):81-88.
40. Eder C. Ion channels in microglia (brain macrophages). Am J Physiol 1998; 275(2 Pt 1):C327-C342.
41. Ilschner S, Ohlemeyer C, Gimpl G et al. Modulation of potassium currents in cultured murine microglial cells by receptor activation and intracellular pathways. Neuroscience 1995; 66(4):983-1000.
42. Fischer HG, Eder C, Hadding U et al. Cytokine-dependent K⁺ channel profile of microglia at immunologically defined functional states. Neuroscience 1995; 64(1):183-191.
43. Schlichter L, Sidell N, Hagiwara S. Potassium channels mediate killing by human natural killer cells. Proc Natl Acad Sci USA 1986; 83(2):451-455.
44. Küst B, Buttini M, Sauter A et al. K⁺-channels and cytokines as markers for microglial activation. Adv Exp Med Biol 1997; 429:109-117.
45. Chung S, Jung W, Lee MY. Inward and outward rectifying potassium currents set membrane potentials in activated rat microglia. Neurosci Lett 1999; 262(2):121-124.
46. McCloskey MA, Qian YX. Selective expression of potassium channels during mast cell differentiation. J Biol Chem 1994; 269:14813-14819.

47. Maltsev VA, Wobus AM, Rohwedel J et al. Cardiomyocytes differentiated in vitro from embryonic stem cells developmentally express cardiac-specific genes and ionic currents. Circ Res 1994; 75:233-244.
48. Shin KS, Park J, Kwon J et al. A possible role of inwardly rectifying K+ channels in chick myoblast differentiation. Am J Physiol 1997; 272 (Cell Physiol 41):C894-C900.
49. Hu Q, Shi YL. Characterization of an inwardly rectifying potassium current in NG108-15 neuroblastoma x glioma cells. Pflugers Arch 1997; 433:617-625.
50. Gerrity RG. The role of the monocyte in atherogenesis: I. Transition of blood-borne monocytes into foam cells in fatty lesions. Am J Pathol 1981; 103(2):181-190.
51. Lei XJ, Ma AQ, Xi YT et al. Expression of Kir2.1 channel during differentiation of human macrophages into foam cells. Di Yi Jun Yi Da Xue Xue Bao 2005; 25(12):1461-1467.
52. Lei XJ, Ma AQ, Xi YT et al. Inhibition of human macrophage-derived foam cell differentiation by blocking Kv1.3 and kir2.1 channels. Zhong Nan Da Xue Xue Bao Yi Xue Ban 2006; 31(4):493-498.
53. Lei XJ, Ma AQ, Xi YT et al. Inhibitory effects of blocking voltage-dependent potassium channel 1.3 on human monocyte-derived macrophage differentiation into foam cells. Beijing Da Xue Xue Bao 2006; 38(3):257-261.
54. Ypey DL, Clapham DE. Development of a delayed outward-rectifying K+ conductance in cultured mouse peritoneal macrophages. Proc Natl Acad Sci USA 1984; 81(10):3083-3087.
55. Chung S, Joe E, Soh H et al. Delayed rectifier potassium currents induced in activated rat microglia set the resting membrane potential. Neurosci Lett 1998; 242(2):73-76.
56. Visentin S, Agresti C, Patrizio M et al. Ion channels in rat microglia and their different sensitivity to lipopolysaccharide and interferon-gamma. J Neurosci Res 1995; 42(4):439-451.
57. Sievers J, Schmidtmayer J, Parwaresch R. Blood monocytes and spleen macrophages differentiate into microglia-like cells when cultured on astrocytes. Ann Anat 1994; 176(1):45-51.
58. Ince C, Coremans JM, Ypey DL et al. Phagocytosis by human macrophages is accompanied by changes in ionic channel currents. J Cell Biol 1988; 106(6):1873-1878.
59. Pannasch U, Färber K, Nolte C et al. The potassium channels Kv1.5 and Kv1.3 modulate distinct functions of microglia. Mol Cell Neurosci 2006; 33(4):401-411. Epub, 2006.
60. Nutile-McMenemy N, Elfenbein A, DeLo JA. Minocycline decreases in vitro microglial motility, β_1-integrin and Kv1.3 channel expression. J Neurochem 2007; 103:2035-2046.
61. Vicente R, Escalada A, Soler C et al. Pattern of kv beta subunit expression in macrophages depends upon proliferation and the mode of activation. J Immunol 2005; 174(8):4736-4744.
62. Vicente R, Escalada A, Villalonga N et al. Association of kv1.5 and kv1.3 contributes to the major voltage-dependent K+ channel in macrophages. J Biol Chem 2006; 281(49):37675-37685. Epub, 2006.
63. Vicente R, Villalonga N, Calvo M et al. Kv1.5 association modifies kv1.3 traffic and membrane localization. J Biol Chem 2008; 283(13):8756-8764. Epub, 2008.
64. Villalonga N, Escalada A, Vicente R et al. Kv1.3/kv1.5 heteromeric channels compromise pharmacological responses in macrophages. Biochem Biophys Res Commun 2007; 352(4):913-918. Epub, 2006.
65. Elbashir SM, Harborth J, Lendeckel W et al. Duplexes of 21-nucleotide RNAs mediate RNA interference in cultured mammalian cells. Nature 2001; 24; 411(6836):494-498.
66. Elbashir SM, Lendeckel W, Tuschl T. RNA interference is mediated by 21- and 22-nucleotide RNAs. Genes Dev 2001; 15(2):188-200.
67. Feral CC, Neels JG, Kummer C et al. Blockade of α4 integrin signaling ameliorates the metabolic consequences of high fat diet-induced obesity. Diabetes 2008; 57(7):1842-1851.

Chapter 9

Integrin Receptors and Ligand-Gated Channels

Raffaella Morini and Andrea Becchetti*

Abstract

Plastic expression of different integrin subunits controls the different stages of neural development, whereas in the adult integrins regulate synaptic stability. Evidence of integrin-channel crosstalk exists for ionotropic glutamate receptors. As is often the case in other tissues, integrin engagement regulates channel activity through complex signaling pathways that often include tyrosine phosphorylation cascades. The specific pathways recruited by integrin activation depend on cerebral region and cell type. In turn, ion channels control integrin expression onto the plasma membrane and their ligand binding affinity. The most extensive studies concern the hippocampus and suggest implications for neuronal circuit plasticity. The physiological relevance of these findings depends on whether adhesion molecules, aside from determining tissue stability, contribute to synaptogenesis and the responsiveness of mature synapses, thus contributing to long term circuit consolidation. Little evidence is available for other ligand-gated channels, with the exception of nicotinic receptors. These exert a variety of functions in neurons and non neural tissue, both in development and in the adult, by regulating cell cycle, synaptogenesis and synaptic circuit refinement. Detailed studies in epidermal keratinocytes have shed some light on the possible mechanisms through which ACh can regulate cell motility, which may be of general relevance for morphogenetic processes. As to the control of mature synapses, most results concern the integrinic control of nicotinic receptors in the neuromuscular junction. Following this lead, a few studies have addressed similar topics in adult cerebral synapses. However, pursuing and interpreting these results in the brain is especially difficult because of the complexity of the nicotinic roles and the widespread contribution of nonsynaptic, paracrine transmission. From a pathological point of view, considering the well-known contribution of both integrins and ligand-gated channels to synaptogenesis and neural regeneration, the above studies point to interesting implications for epileptogenesis.

Introduction

Integrin receptors are a major family of αβ heterodimeric surface glycoproteins that mediate cell-cell and cell-matrix adhesion. Eighteen α subunits and eight β subunits are presently known, which makes the formation of over 20 dimer combinations possible.[1] Integrins transduce signals bidirectionally between the external environment and the intracellular cytoskeleton and signaling machinery. Thus, they have both "inside out" and "outside in" signaling functions.[2,3] A variety of stimuli target the cytoplasmic integrin domain. The ensuing conformational changes propagate to the extracellular domain and stimulate the ligand binding activity (receptor's 'activation'). In

---

*Corresponding Author: Andrea Becchetti—Department of Biotechnology and Biosciences, University of Milano-Bicocca, Piazza della Scienza 2, 20126 Milano, Italy. Email: andrea.becchetti@unimib.it

Integrins and Ion Channels: Molecular Complexes and Signaling, edited by Andrea Becchetti and Annarosa Arcangeli. ©2010 Landes Bioscience and Springer Science+Business Media.

turn, ligand binding affects the physical arrangement of integrin-associated cytoskeletal proteins[4] as well as regulatory elements comprising the focal adhesion kinase (FAK), the Src family kinase fyn, MAP kinase, protein phosphatases and PI(3) kinase, to name a few. In this way, integrin ligand binding stimulates cytoplasmic tyrosine phosphorylation cascades such as the Ras/Raf/MEK/ERK pathway, ultimately producing a modulatory feedback on integrin properties and expression.[5]

Most of what is known about the relations between ligand-gated channels and integrin receptors concerns the mammalian brain. In the following, we summarize current knowledge on the differential distribution and roles of integrin receptors in the developing and adult brain, with special attention to the cerebral cortex. Early studies date back to the 1980s. More recently, a wealth of information about the integrin roles in neural development has come from gene deletion approaches, mostly carried out by producing knockout murine strains.

Much of the initial interest in integrin functions in the nervous system focused on the neural crest, a migratory cell population derived from the dorsal neural tube. Neural crest cells express many integrin types that mediate and regulate their migration through a matrix-rich environment, steadily and abundantly coated by fibronectin and laminin, for example.[6,7] In the cerebral cortex, α3β1 interaction with reelin, an extracellular matrix protein (ECM) released from cortical neurons, is thought to be a crucial step in the appropriate placement of neurons in developing layers.[8] An elegant work of Graus-Porta and colleagues showed that β1 deletion, which results in the ablation of about ten integrin types, produces severe brain abnormalities.[9] Surprisingly, however, neurons can still form adhesive interaction with the radial glia fibers. They thus migrate normally along the fibers and take up their appropriate positions in layers. In fact, conspicuous disorganization was only observed in the most superficial layer of the cortex, the marginal zone. Therefore, the defects in cortical foliation and lamination in β1 deficient mice arise mainly as a consequence of perturbations in the cortical marginal zone. Recent results further clarified the role of β1-containing integrins, by showing that α3β1 is required for glial (but not neuronal) migration, whereas it is involved in both glial and neuronal maturation.[10] Other integrin types, such as αv and α6 have been found to be necessary for cerebral cortex development, since distinct and severe cortical malformations were observed in murine strains knocked out for these proteins.[11]

The cerebral expression of integrins is continuously changing during development because it follows the expression of different ECM environments in the different stages. Some forms however do persist in the adult brain, where in situ hybridization analyses show highly specific regional patterns in the expression of integrin expression, at least in the rat.[12] Of the β integrins, β1, β3 and β5 are found throughout the developing cerebral wall and persist in the adult, particularly in the hippocampal and cortical synapses. The same applies to β8, which is however also expressed in glial cells. The other β's are only expressed in the adult. In particular, β2 and β4 are confined to the hippocampus, whereas β6 is detected in both cerebral cortex and hippocampus.[13,14]

As to the α integrins, α1, α3 and α4 are widely distributed in the developing rat brain, whereas in the adult their expression is confined to a few specific layers in the hippocampus, cerebellum and neocortex. In contrast, α5 and α7 integrins are found exclusively in the adult brain, especially on neocortical cell bodies and apical dendrites.[12] More detailed morphological studies are available for α8, which appears in cortical neuron dendrites as early as embryonic day 16. This subunit has been localized by electron microscopy to the dendritic spines of hippocampal pyramidal neurons and granule cells, where it is associated with the postsynaptic densities. Finally, αv expression is observed in the radial glial fibers of the developing cerebral cortex and persists in neurons and astrocytes of the mature cortex. The distribution of integrin subunits in the rat brain is summarized in Table 1.

The Functional Significance of Integrins in the Adult Brain

As briefly illustrated above, many integrins are localized specifically at synapses (in particular α3, α5, α8, αv and β1, β3, β8). Recent physiological and functional observations support the idea that this family of adhesion molecules, far from simply determining neural tissue stability, contribute to synaptogenesis and the physiology of mature synapses, often through the mediation of ion channel modulation.

Table 1. Distribution of integrin subunits in rat cerebral cortex and hippocampus

	α1	α2	α3	α4	α5	α6	α7	α8	αV	β1	β2	β3	β4	β5	β6	β7	β8
Developing cerebral wall	+	–	+	+	–	+	–	+	+	+	–	+	–	+	–	–	+
Adult brain																	
Neocortical layers	5	–	2-6	2-3	2-6	6	2-6	5-6	2-6	1-6	–	+	–	1-5	1-6	–	1-6
Hippocampus	+	–	+	+	+	–	+	+	+	+	+	+	+	+	+	–	+
Cell types																	
Neurons	+	–	+	+	+	–	+	+	+	+	–	+	–	+	+	–	+
Oligodendroglia	–	–	–	–	–	–	–	–	–	–	–	–	–	–	–	–	+
Astrocytes	+	–	–	–	+	–	–	–	+	–	–	–	–	–	–	–	+
Localized at synapse	+	–	+	–	+	–	–	+	+	+	–	+	–	–	–	–	+

Table summarizes data from references 11-14.

Integrin and Ion Channels in Remodeling Adult Circuits and Epileptogenesis

In the adult CNS, integrin receptors are implicated in neural regeneration, synaptogenesis and epileptogenesis. Studies on dissociated hippocampal neurons in primary cultures suggest that integrins mediate the stimulating effect of astrocytes on excitatory synaptogenesis. In particular, integrin-dependent astrocyte-neuron adhesion locally activates protein kinase C (PKC). Such a focal activation is subsequently relayed from the adhesion site and facilitates synaptogenesis throughout the neuron.[15] What is more, integrin receptors regulate the maturation of hippocampal synapses. In early development, N-methyl-D-aspartate glutamate receptors (NMDAR) consist primarily of NR2B subunits, whereas NR2A expression is turned on at a later stage. Such a subunit switch is considered a postsynaptic maturation marker. It is prevented by chronic treatment with the RGD peptide, which mimics ECM protein adhesion to integrin receptors, or by applying specific antibodies against the β3 integrin subunit. Because β3 forms heterodimers exclusively with αIIB or αv and because only the latter is expressed in the brain, αvβ3 heterodimers turn out to be necessary for maturation of excitatory synapses.[16] Integrins containing β1 were also found to be required at an early stage, where they control the maturation of the releasable pool of presynaptic vesicles. In their absence, the synaptic capability of releasing docked vescicles appears to be permanently impaired.[17]

Considering the roles of integrins in neuronal circuit maturation and ion channel regulation, it is not surprising that they have been also implicated in epileptogenetic processes. Seizures and sub-seizure neuronal activity modulate integrins, the expression of matrix ligands and the activity of the proteases that regulate both. Interestingly, seizures induced by pharmacological and electrical stimulation prompts expression of the tissue plasminogen activator (tPA) gene throughout the brain and particularly in the hippocampus.[18] tPA is an extracellular serine protease that converts the inactive integrin ligand plasminogen to the active protease plasmin. The activated tPA-plasmin system turned out to induce mossy fiber sprouting and regulate the level of laminin during neuronal death in the hippocampus.[19,20] Therefore, the interplay of altered neuronal activity, extracellular matrix and integrin function appears to be involved in the complex control of neuronal cell death, axonal regeneration and sprouting, with the consequent development of aberrant innervation patterns which may underlie some forms of epileptic activity. For further review on integrins and epileptogenesis, see ref. 21.

Integrins and Synaptic Plasticity

As suggested by recent work, synaptic glutamate receptors are often activated by integrins, which clearly presents implications for synaptic plasticity in the CNS. The potential integrin function in mediating some of the anatomical and physiological aspects of neuronal plasticity was first suggested by Lynch and colleagues, based on studies where inhibitors of integrin-mediated adhesion blocked long-term potentiation (LTP) in adult rat slices.[22]

LTP stabilization is also effectively inhibited by injection of certain snake toxins (disintegrins), which preferentially inhibit the β1- and β3-mediated binding processes,[23] whereas specific blocking antibodies against α3 facilitate the reversal of LTP.[24] Consistently, mice with reduced expression of α3, α5 and α8 integrin subunits are defective in LTP and spatial memory in the CA1 region of hippocampus, although they respond normally to fear conditioning.[25] In particular, specific knockout of α3 integrin in murine excitatory neurons impairs LTP at the synapses between Schaffer collaterals and the CA1 region. Behavioral studies indicate that the effects on LTP and working memory are similar to those observed in β1-integrin conditional knockout mice. Hence, the α3β1 heterodimer (profusely expressed in central synapses) and its interaction with laminin may be one of the functional cues necessary to develop this particular type of memory.[26,27] More detailed information about the dynamics of integrin intervention in LTP consolidation has come from using specific antibodies locally perfused in hippocampal fields, at different times after LTP induction by theta burst stimulation. These experiments have pointed especially to α3β1 and α5β1. Differently from the results obtained with the broad spectrum RGD peptide, this method permits a dissection of the time course of integrin action and suggests the interesting possibility that LTP comprises more than one integrin-dependent consolidation stage.[23]

From a mechanistic point of view, it appears that β1 integrin selectively controls both actin polymerization and LTP stabilization, suggesting that it regulates the spine actin changes that accompany LTP.[28] It remains however to be understood how integrins could enhance and stabilize long term potentiation. Little conclusive evidence is available to date and different hypotheses, not mutually exclusive, have been advanced. Integrins could control the intracellular Ca^{2+} concentration. It is also possible that tetanic stimulation induces integrin clustering or the formation of integrin-channel complexes with consequent channel and thus synaptic, modulation. Some or all of these effects could depend on integrin-dependent regulation of the protein kinases involved in LTP as well as those which phosphorylate glutamate receptors. These putative mechanisms provide possible links between integrin signaling and the events that express and stabilize LTP. In the following, we describe in more details what is known about the interplay between neuronal glutamate receptors and integrin receptors. The crosstalk between integrins and glutamate receptors in other systems such as T-cells have been reviewed elsewhere.[29]

Integrins and NMDA Receptors

Studies carried out in rat hippocampal slices and synaptoneurosomes show that integrin engagement with GRGDSP, a peptide analogous to RGD, leads to potentiation of NMDA-gated currents, in mature synapses.[30,31] Because paired-pulse facilitation is unaffected, integrin activation does not seem to modify GABAergic transmission or, in general, neurotransmitter release. The stimulation produced by GRGDSP depends on tyrosine phosphorylation pathways, since it is abolished by inhibiting Src kinase. Recent work refines this scheme and leads to attribute these effects to potent activation of FAK and the associated protein Pyk2, with ensuing Src kinase-dependent phosphorylation of both NR2A and NR2B channel subunits.[31]

NMDAR recruitment suggests that integrin signaling could affect Ca^{2+}-dependent signaling, with possible ensuing long-term nuclear effects. This has been confirmed by applying both imaging and biochemical experiments on neurons dissociated from the rat neocortex.[32] GRGDSP perfusion stimulates Ca^{2+} influx from the extracellular medium, which is abolished by inhibiting the NMDA channels. This process is accompanied by phosphorylation and nuclear traslocation of ERK1/2, mediated by Src and MAP kinase activation. However, in these neurons the GRGDSP-mediated activation of the ERK1/2 kinase pathway does not depend on any typical mediator of integrin signaling. No phosphorylation is observed on Tyr-397 of FAK, nor any modification is observed in Ca^{2+}-calmodulin dependent protein kinase II (CaMKII).[32] Hence, in the brain, not only integrin subunit expression, but also the signaling pathways recruited by integrin-mediated adhesion depend on the cerebral region and the cell type where integrins operate.

Integrins and AMPA Receptors

Once again, most of the evidence concerns rat hippocampal slices, where perfusion of GRGDSP reversibly increases the slope and amplitude of the fast excitatory postsynaptic potentials (fEPSPs), because of α-amino-3-hydroxy-5-methyl-4-isoxazolepropionic acid receptor (AMPAR) activation.[33] This response is inhibited by application of a mixture of antibodies against α3, α5 and αv and is accompanied by phosphorylation of CaMKII and the GluR1 subunit of AMPARs. Synaptic potentiation is blocked when inhibitors of NMDARs and Src kinase are applied together. On the other hand, to inhibit the two phosphorylation steps, it is sufficient to block the NMDA channels. Therefore, integrin engagement must activate at least two different pathways. One of them is Src-independent and leads to NMDA current stimulation, with ensuing CaMKII and GluR1 phosphorylation, which leads to AMPAR potentiation. A second pathway is mediated by Src-kinase activation and also modulates, directly or indirectly, the AMPARs.[33] Complementary studies have been carried out by using β1 integrin knockout mice. In these, fEPSPs at CA3-CA1 synapses are dramatically reduced, most probably because postsynaptic

AMPAR are defective.[26] Irrespective of the details, these results show that hippocampal integrin activation is necessary to control the functional level of postsynaptic AMPARs.

Very recent work has begun to address the effect of integrin activation in the cerebral cortex, by using neuron-enriched primary neocortical cultures.[34] Treatment with RGD or α5β1-activating antisera produces a rapid and prolonged increase in $[Ca^{2+}]_i$. This response was reduced by inhibiting the voltage-sensitive Ca^{2+} channels and the NMDARs, but completely blocked only by concomitant application of tetrodoxin and antagonists of AMPARs and tyrosine kinases. Therefore, in cortical pyramidal neurons, integrin activation stimulates the AMPARs through recruitment of tyrosine kinase pathways. As a consequence, a massive Ca^{2+} influx is triggered, through different pathways both voltage-dependent and independent, such as voltage-gated Ca^{2+} channels, NMDARs, release from intracellular stores, etc.

As is the case for other ion channels, it is clear that the crosstalk between integrins and AMPARs is intricate and includes feedback from channel activation to integrin expression. In particular, channel activity stimulates the membrane expression of α5 and β1 subunits. Once inserted into the plasma membrane, these subunits activate and produce stimulation of kinase-dependent signaling.[35] These studies provide nice examples of the typical bidirectional signaling between integrin receptors and ion channels.[2,3,29] Integrins modulate channel function mostly through tyrosine kinase activation, whereas ion channels control either integrin expression onto the plasma membrane or their ligand binding affinity. A summary of the signaling network connecting integrin receptors and ionotropic glutamate receptors is given in Figure 1.

Integrins and GABA Receptors: Further Possibilities to Modulate Synaptic Plasticity?

Neuronal liability to LTP development could also be regulated by modulation of inhibitory synapses and at least one study suggests that integrin activation may produce such an effect. When properly stimulated, the GABAergic synapses onto cerebellar Purkinje neurons show a long-term potentiation of $GABA_A$ responsiveness (called rebound potentiation). This process is impaired when integrins are activated by Mn^{2+}, with consequent inhibition of the miniature IPSCs at Purkinje neurons. The effect depends on α3 and β1 integrins and is mediated by the Src-family PTK activity.[36] Because it is unclear whether α3β1 is expressed on GABAergic neurons, it is possible that integrins modulate GABAergic currents indirectly. Nonetheless, this example shows that integrin activation can contribute to control synaptic plasticity at inhibitory synapses.

Integrins and Nicotinic Acetylcholine Receptors: Not Only the Neuromuscular Junction

Studies in Nonneural Tissue

Cholinergic signaling appears very early in development. ACh regulates cell division and motility since gastrulation, but nAChRs have been detected even at earlier stages, such as sea urchin oocytes and appear to play functional roles well before neuronal differentiation.[37,38] In fact, nicotinic subunit expression precedes that of other ligand-gated channels as well as the one of muscarinic receptors. At these early stages, nAChRs contribute to regulate as different processes as cell cycle, apoptosis, neuronal differentiation and guidance of nerve growth cones. For review, see ref 39. In later phases, they participate to the refinement of neuronal networks. In the rodent's forebrain and cortex, an upsurge of nAChR expression occurs during the first two weeks of postnatal development, when the ascending cholinergic projections invade the neocortex.[40,41]

Nicotinic expression persists in the adult, with physiological roles that are only beginning to be understood. Studies in human epidermal keratinocytes, in particular, have shed some light on the mechanisms through which ACh regulates cell motility, which may be of general relevance. These cells synthesize and secrete ACh, which controls several functions, including motility, in a paracrine way.[42] Concerted activation of α7 nAChRs and muscarinic M1 receptors

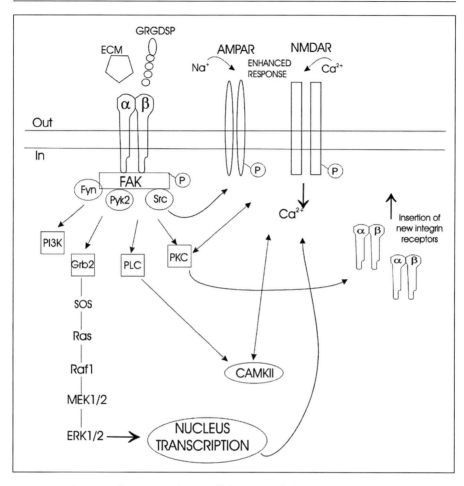

Figure 1. Schematic illustration of intracellular crosstalk between integrins and glutamate receptors in brain. As described in text, integrin activation leads to increase in synaptic glutamatergic responses through several tyrosine kinase activation. In turn, ion channel activity can control integrin expression onto the plasma membrane. Figure summarizes data from references 30-33, 35.

leads to engage the Ras/Raf1/MEK1/ERK signaling pathway that, in turn, up-regulates the expression of α2 and α3 Integrins. Thus, α7 nAChRs cooperate with muscarinic receptors to orient keratinocytes towards its future migration path by increasing the expression of α2 and α3 integrins required to stabilize the lamellipodium.[43] These mechanisms are further discussed in Chapter 10.

Another issue that may be of general importance is the cholinergic regulation of cell division in preneural embryos, which points to a widespread nAChR role in cell cycle control. Other sections of the present book illustrate how integrins and ion channels interact in the multiple steps of neoplastic progression. Here, we notice that these ideas may also apply to nAChRs. Nicotine has been recently found to stimulate human lung cancer cell growth by inducing fibronectin expression, which also offers interesting hints about nicotine long-term harmful effects.[44] In brief, in cultured nonsmall cell lung carcinoma, nicotine stimulates membrane expression of α7 nAChRs as well as fibronectin production. The nicotine-induced fibronectin response and the ensuing cell proliferation are abolished by α-bungarotoxin, an inhibitor of α7 nAChR. Cell proliferation is also inhibited by using an antibody against the α5β1 integrin, which binds fibronectin in normal conditions. Therefore, nicotine stimulates nonsmall cell lung carcinoma proliferation in a way mediated by a fibronectin induction, which is dependent on α7 nAChR activation. As is also the case for other integrin-dependent signals associated with ion channel activation, the nAChR-mediated signals appear to include the ERK and PI3-K/mTOR pathways.[44]

Studies in the Neuromuscular Junction and the Central Nervous System

The best characterized example of interaction between integrin receptors and nAChRs is the ECM-dependent nAChRs clustering at the neuromuscular junction (NMJ), which is a critical step in neuromuscular synaptogenesis.[45] This process is induced by laminin and agrin, which probably activate different signaling pathways. A specific isoform of α7β1 integrin has been observed to colocalize and physically interact with clustered nAChRs in a laminin-dependent manner.[46] Cell adhesion to laminin induces tyrosine phosphorylation on the β1 subunit of the nAChR, which appears to be necessary for nAChR clustering and complex stabilization.[47]

Are the above observations relevant for synaptic physiology in the CNS? Agrin and laminin are widely expressed in the brain. Recent work in vivo shows that agrin is required for functional development of interneuronal synapses. It also suggests a novel role for agrin in stabilizing the postsynaptic density of nAChR at nascent synapses.[48] Agrin signaling in neocortical neurons involve tyrosine kinases, CaMKII and the MAPK signal pathways.[49] Whether integrins are involved in these processes is unknown. More generally, transferring knowledge obtained from studies on NMJ and glutamate receptors to cerebral nAChRs is not straightforward, because of the special features of cholinergic transmission in the brain. The ascending cholinergic system targets both nicotinic and muscarinic receptors in the cerebral cortex, thalamus and other regions. In this way, it regulates vigilance and the transitions between different cerebral states, such as the non rapid eye movement and the rapid eye movement phases of sleep.[50] In particular, nAChRs are expressed throughout the brain and contribute to these and other functions, such as the regulation of synaptic transmission and synaptic plasticity, particularly in the hippocampus, with a variety of cognitive implications.[51] Usually, nicotinic activation leads to membrane depolarization and, depending on receptor's type, to variable levels of Ca^{2+} influx, with possible ensuing activation of intracellular signaling mechanisms and gene transcription (see Chapter 2). The special complexity of nicotinic transmission is caused by the nAChR expression at presynaptic, postsynaptic and preterminal level. What is more, cholinergic innervation in the brain prevalently (but not exclusively) shows a diffuse nature, with ACh probably often exerting paracrine transmission.[52,53] Therefore, the nAChR interactions with the extracellular matrix should present very interesting peculiarities and knowledge obtained from glutamatergic transmission may not be directly relevant.

Conclusion

From a pathological standpoint, the nAChR relations with ECM seems worth deepening because of the nAChR role during synapse pruning and by analogy with the epileptogenic implications suggested by work on glutamate receptors. Interestingly, nAChRs are sensitive to mutation, in terms of epileptogenic potential, differently from glutamate receptors.[54] A number of dominant mutations on α4, β2 and α2 nAChR subunit genes are linked to certain sleep-related epileptic forms, arising in the frontal lobes.[55-58] When expressed in heterologous systems, these mutations produce different degrees of functional alteration, whose pathogenetic meaning is still unclear. Subtle differences in channel structure and function may affect channel interaction with the ECM and synapse formation in critical stages, with possible epileptogenic effects that are still totally unexplored.

Acknowledgements

This work has been supported by grants from the Italian Ministry of University and Scientific Research, the University of Milano-Bicocca (FAR) and the Fondazione Banca del Monte Lombardia.

References

1. Humphries MJ, Delwel GO, Kuikman I et al. Integrin structure. Biochem Soc Trans 2000; 28:311-339.
2. Hynes RO. Integrins: bidirectional, allosteric signaling machines. Cell 2002; 110:673-687.
3. Mould AP. Getting integrins into shape: recent insights into how integrin activity is regulated by conformational changes. J Cell Sci 1996; 109:2613-2618.
4. Dedhar S, Hanningan G. Integrin cytoplasmic interaction and bidirectional transmembrane signaling. Curr Opin Cell Biol 1996; 8:657-669.
5. Juliano RL. Signal transduction by cell adhesion receptors and the cytoskeleton: functions of integrins, cadherins, selectins and immunoglobulin-superfamily members. Annu Rev Pharmacol Toxicol 2002; 42:283-323.
6. Bronner-Fraser M. Neural crest cell formation and migration in the developing embryo. FASEB J 1994; 8:699-706.
7. Kil SH, Krull CE, Cann G et al. The alpha4 subunit of integrin is important for neural cell crest migration. Dev Biol 1998; 202:29-42.
8. Schmid RS, Jo R, Shelton S et al. Reelin, integrin and DAB1 interaction during embryonic cerebral cortical development. Cereb Cortex 2005; 15:1632-1636.
9. Graus-Porta D, Blaess S, Senften M et al. β1-class integrin regulate the development of laminae and folia in the cerebral and cerebellar cortex. Neuron 2001; 31:367-379.
10. Belvindrah R, Graus-Porta D, Goebbels S et al. Beta1 integrins in radial glia but not in migrating neurons are essential for the formation of cell layers in the cerebral cortex. J Neurosci 2007; 27:13854-13865.
11. Schmid RS, Anton ES. Role of integrins in the development of the cerebral cortex. Cereb Cortex 2003; 13:219-224.
12. Pinkstaff JK, Detterich J, Lynch G et al. Integrin subunit gene expression is regionally differentiated in adult brain. J Neurosci 1999; 19:1541-1556.
13. Nishimura SL, Boylen KP, Einheber S et al. Synaptic and glial localization of the integrin alphavbeta8 in mouse and rat brain. Brain Res 1998; 791:271-282.
14. Cousin B, Leloup C, Penicaud L et al. Developmental changes in integrin beta-subunits in rat cerebral cortex. Neurosci Lett 1997; 234:161-165.
15. Hama H, Hara C, Yamaguchi K et al. PKC signalling mediates global enhancement of excitatory synaptogenesis in neurons triggered by local contact with astrocytes. Neuron 2004; 41:405-415.
16. Chavis P, Westbrook G. Integrins mediate functional pre and postsynaptic maturation at a hippocampal synapse. Nature 2001; 411:317-321.
17. Huang Z, Shimazu K, Wu NH et al. Distict roles of beta1-class of integrins at the developing and the mature hippocampal excitatory synapse. J Neurosci 2006; 26:11208-11219.
18. Quan A, Gilbert M, Colicos M et al. Tissue-plasminogen activator is induced as an immediate-early gene during seizure, kindling and long-term potentiation. Nature 1993; 361:453-457.
19. Wu YP, Siao CJ, Lu W et al. The tissue plasminogen activator (tPA)/plasmin extracellular proteolytic system regulates seizure-induced hippocampal mossy fiber outgrowth through a proteoglycan substrate. J Cell Biochem 2000; 148:1295-1304.
20. Chen A L, Strickland S. Neuronal death in hippocampus is promoted by plasmin-catalyzed degradation of laminin. Cell 1997; 91:917-925.
21. Gall CM, Lynch G. Integrins, synaptic plasticity and epileptogenesis. Adv Exp Med Biol 2004; 548:12-33.
22. Staubli U, Vanderklish P, Lynch G. An inhibitor of integrin receptors blocks long-term potentiation. Behav Neural Biol 1990; 53:1-5.
23. Chun D, Gall CM, Bi X et al. Evidence that integrins contribute to multiple stages in the consolidation of long term potentiation in rat hippocampus. Neurosci 2001; 105:815-829.
24. Kramar EA, Bernard JA, Gall CM et al. Alpha3 integrin receptors contribute to the consolidation of long-term potentiation. Neurosci 2002; 110:29-39.
25. Chan CS, Weeber EJ, Kurup S et al. Integrin requirement for hippocampal synaptic plasticity and spatial memory. J Neurosci 2003; 23:7107-7116.

26. Chan CS, Weeber EJ, Zong L et al. Beta1-integrins are required for hippocampal AMPA receptor dependent synaptic transmission, synaptic plasticity and working memory. J Neurosci 2006; 26:223-232.
27. Chan CS, Levenson JM, Mukhopadhyay PS et al. Alpha3-integrins are required for hippocampal long-term potentiation and working memory. Learn Mem 2007; 14:606-615.
28. Kramar EA, Lin B, Rex CS et al. Integrin-driven actin polymerization consolidates long-term potentiation. Proc Natl Acad Sci USA 2006; 103:5579-5584.
29. Arcangeli A, Becchetti A. Complex functional interaction between integrin receptors and ion channels. Trends Cell Biol 2006; 16:631-63931.
30. Lin B, Arai AC, Lynch G et al. Integrins regulate NMDA receptor-mediated synaptic currents. J Neurophysiol 2003; 89:2874-2878.
31. Bernard-Trifilo JA, Kramar AE, Torp R et al. Integrin signaling cascades are operational in adult hippocampal synapses and modulate NMDA receptor physiology. J Neurochem 2005; 93:834-849.
32. Watson PMD, Humphries MJ, Relton J et al. Integrin-binding RGD peptides induce rapid intracellular calcium increases and MAPK signaling in cortical neurons. Mol Cell Neurosci 2007; 34:147-154.
33. Kramar EA, Bernard JA, Gall CM et al. Integrins modulate fast synaptic transmission at hippocampal synapses. J Biol Chem 2003; 278:10722-10730.
34. Lin C-Y, Hilgenberg LG, Smith MA et al. Integrin regulation of cytoplasmic calcium in excitatory neurons depends upon glutamate receptors and release from intracellular stores. Mol Cell Neurosci 2008; 37:770-780.
35. Lin C-Y, Lynch G, Gall CM. AMPA receptor stimulation increases alpha5beta1 integrin surface expression, adhesive function and signaling. J Neurochem 2005; 94:531-546.
36. Kawaguchi SY, Hirano T. Integrin alpha3beta1 suppresses long-term potentiation at inhibitory synapses on the cerebellar Purkinje neuron. Mol Cell Neurosci 2006; 31:416-426.
37. Smith J, Fauquet M, Ziller C et al. Acetylcholine synthesis by mesencephalic neural crest cells in the process of migration in vivo. Nature 1979; 282:853-855.
38. Buznikov GA, Shmukler YB, Lauder JM. From oocyte to neuron: do neurotransmitters function in the same way throughout development? Cell Mol Neurobiol 1996; 16:537-559.
39. Mansvelder HD, Role LW. Neuronal receptors for nicotine: functional diversity and developmental changes. In brain development. Normal processes and the effects of alcohol and nicotine. Oxford University Press, 2006.
40. Fuchs JL. (^{125}I)α-bungarotoxin binding marks primary sensory area developing rat neocortex. Brain Res 1989; 501:223-234.
41. Broide RS, Robertson RT, Leslie FM. Regulation of α7 nicotinic acetylcholine receptors in the developing rat somatosensory cortex by thalamocortical afferents. J Neurosci 1996; 16:2956-2971.
42. Grando SA, Horton RM, Pereira EF et al. A nicotinic acetylcholine receptor regulating cell adhesion and motility is expressed in human keratinocytes. J Invest Dermatol 1995; 107:774-771.
43. Chernyavsky AI, Arredondo J, Karlsson E et al. The Ras/Raf-1/MEK1/ERK signaling pathway coupled to integrin expression mediates cholinergic regulation of keratinocyte directional migration. J Biol Chem 2005; 280:39220-39228.
44. Zhen Y, Ritzenthaler JD, Roman J et al. Nicotine stimulates human lung cancer cell growth by inducing fibronectin expression. Am J Respir Cell Mol Biol 2007; 37:681-690.
45. Willmann R, Fuhrer C. Neuromuscular synaptogenesis: clustering of acetylcholine receptors revisited. Cell Mol Life Sci 2002; 59:1296-1316.
46. Burkin JD, Kim JE, Gu M et al. Laminin and α7β1 integrin regulate agrin-induced clustering of acetylcholine receptors. J Cell Sci 2000; 113:2877-2886.
47. Marangi PA, Weland ST, Fuhrer C. Laminin-1 redistributes postsynaptic proteins and requires rapsyn, tyrosine phosphorylation and Src and Fyn to stably cluster acetylcholine receptors. J Cell Biol 2002; 157:883-895.
48. Gingras J, Rassadi S, Cooper E et al. Synaptic transmission is impaired at neuronal autonomic synapses in agrin-null mice. Dev Neurobiol 2007; 67:521-534.
49. Hilgenberg LG, Smith MA. Agrin signaling in cortical neurons is mediated by a tyrosine kinase-dependent increase in intracellular Ca^{2+} that engages both CaMKII and MAPK signal pathways. J Neurobiol 2004; 61:289-300.
50. Steriade M, McCarley R. Brain control of wakefulness and sleep. 2nd Ed. Plenum Publishers, 2005.
51. McKey BE, Placzek AN, Dani JA. Regulation of synaptic transmission and plasticity by neuronal nicotinic acetylcholine receptors. Biochem Pharmacol 2007; 74:1120-1133.
52. Zoli M, Jansson A, Sykova E et al. Volume transmission in the CNS and its relevance for neuropsychopharmacology. Trends Pharmacol 1999; 20:142-150.

53. Mechawar N, Watkins KC, Descarries L. Ultrastructural features of the acetylcholine innervation in the developing parietal cortex of rat. J Comp Neurol 2002; 443:250-258.
54. Helbig I, Scheffer IE, Mulley JC et al. Navigating the channels and beyond: unravelling the genetics of the epilepsies. Lancet Neurol 2008; 7:231-245.
55. Steinlein OK, Mulley JC, Propping P et al. A missense mutation in the neuronal nicotinic acetylcholine receptor alfa4 subunit is associated with autosomal dominant nocturnal frontal lobe epilepsy. Nat Genet 1995; 11:201-203.
56. De Fusco M, Becchetti A, Patrignani M et al. The nicotinic receptor beta 2 subunit is mutant in nocturnal frontal lobe epilepsy. Nat Genet 2000; 26:275-276.
57. Phillips HA, Favre I, Kirkpatrick M et al. CHRNB2 is the second acetylcholine receptor subunit associated with autosomal dominant nocturnal frontal lobe epilepsy. Am J Hum Genet 2001; 68:225-231.
58. Aridon P, Marini C, Di Resta C et al. Increased sensitivity of the neuronal nicotinic receptor alpha 2 subunit causes familial epilepsy with nocturnal wandering and ictal fear. Am J Hum Genet 2006; 79:342-350.

CHAPTER 10

Integrins and Ion Channels in Cell Migration:
Implications for Neuronal Development, Wound Healing and Metastatic Spread

Andrea Becchetti* and Annarosa Arcangeli

Abstract

Cell migration is necessary for proper embryonic development and adult tissue remodeling. Its mechanisms determine the physiopathology of processes such as neuronal targeting, inflammation, wound healing and metastatic spread. Crawling of cells onto solid surfaces requires a controlled sequence of cell protrusions and retractions that mainly depends on sophisticated regulation of the actin cytoskeleton, although the contribution of microtubules should not be neglected. This process is triggered and modulated by a combination of diffusible and fixed environmental signals. External cues are sensed and integrated by membrane receptors, including integrins, which transduce these signals into cellular signaling pathways, often centered on the small GTPase proteins belonging to the Rho family. These pathways regulate the coordinated cytoskeletal rearrangements necessary for proper timing of adhesion, contraction and detachment at the front and rear side of cells finding their way through the extracellular spaces. The overall process involves continuous modulation of cell motility, shape and volume, in which ion channels play major roles. In particular, Ca^{2+} signals have both global and local regulatory effects on cell motility, because they target the contractile proteins as well as many regulatory proteins.

After reviewing the fundamental mechanisms of eukaryotic cell migration onto solid substrates, we briefly describe how integrin receptors and ion channels are involved in cell movement. We next examine a few processes in which these mechanisms have been studied in depth. We thus illustrate how integrins and K^+ channels control cell volume and migration, how intracellular Ca^{2+} homeostasis affects the motility of neuronal growth cones and what is known about the ion channel roles in epithelial cell migration. These mechanisms are implicated in a variety of pathological processes, such as the disruption of neural circuits and wound healing.

Finally, we describe the interaction between neoplastic cells and their local environment and how derangement of adhesion can lead to metastatic spread. It is likely that the cellular mechanisms controlled by integrin receptors, ion channels or both participate in the entire metastatic process. Until now, however, evidence is limited to a few steps of the metastatic cascade, such as brain tumor invasiveness.

*Corresponding Author: Andrea Becchetti—Department of Biotechnology and Biosciences, University of Milano-Bicocca, Piazza della Scienza 2, 20126 Milan, Italy. Email: andrea.becchetti@unimib.it

Integrins and Ion Channels: Molecular Complexes and Signaling, edited by Andrea Becchetti and Annarosa Arcangeli. ©2010 Landes Bioscience and Springer Science+Business Media.

Introduction

With the exception of spermatozoa, mammalian cell locomotion occurs by amoeboid movement onto solid surfaces (crawling). Proper cell migration is crucial during development and particularly in the nervous system, where cell motility determines not only neuronal targeting to the final address, but also the subsequent neurite sprouting and synaptic formation. The mechanisms underlying these processes remain active in the adult nervous system, where they control synaptic plasticity and neuronal regeneration. Other examples that have been the object of thorough studies are leukocyte migration towards infection sites, connective tissue remodeling by fibroblasts, tissue renewal and wound healing in epithelia. Even such an incomplete list is immediately suggestive of the great pathological relevance of cell locomotion control. Moreover, derangement of tissue stability and improper activation of cell movement are crucial steps of tumor progression and are implicated in neoplastic cell invasion of healthy tissue, dissemination through blood stream and further invasion of distant sites.

Actin Cytoskeleton

Cell crawling depends on actin filaments (also named microfilaments) highly concentrated in the cell cortex close to the plasma membrane. For reader's convenience, we give an outline of the physiology of actin cytoskeleton. Excellent introductions to the field are found in refs. 1 and 2. Microfilaments are double right-handed helix polymers of non covalently associated globular actin subunits. These can form linear bundles, but also two- or three-dimensional arrays, whose degree of branching and stiffness are controlled by accessory proteins. Actin filaments are polar structures, in that monomers bind head-to-tail to produce filaments bearing two ends with different properties, called *plus* and *minus* end. The former undergoes more rapid assembly-disassembly of subunits, in the presence of ATP. Each monomer contains a binding site for ATP or ADP. Hydrolysis of ATP provides the free energy necessary for filament elongation, which determines the extension of cellular protrusions. At rest, assembly and disassembly at both ends maintain microfilaments at a stable length. In the more stable tissues, specific accessory proteins further decrease the cytoskeletal dynamics. More than a hundred proteins are known to bind actin. Among those implicated in microfilament bundling and cross-linking, we recall fimbrin, α-actinin and filamin. Other proteins control actin attachment to the plasma membrane, e.g., spectrin and the ERM family (from the initials of ezrin, radixin, mesin).[1] During crawling, directional assembly of microfilaments produces oriented movement. Actin nucleation usually occurs near the plasma membrane and is regulated by a variety of extracellular signals, which activate intracellular pathways that generally converge on two types of regulatory proteins: the ARP complex (so called because it includes the actin-related proteins, ARPs) and the formins. ARP binds to the *minus* end of the actin rod and is usually found in cell regions with rapid microfilament growth. It can connect different filaments to form branched structures and typically leads to the nucleation of gel-like three-dimensional networks. Formins are dimeric proteins which can nucleate the formation of new actin filaments, by associating at the *plus* end. They do not allow the formation of branched structures and thus favor the nucleation of cytoskeletal structures made by parallel bundles.[3] Microfilament elongation is also regulated by specific intracellular proteins. Two major competing elements are thymosin, which associates to free actin and blocks the polymerization of monomers and profilin, which instead stimulates polymerization. The balance of these effects is regulated by different intracellular cascades activated by extracellular signals. When needed, the actin cytoskeleton can be efficiently disassembled. A major regulatory protein implicated in microfilament destabilization is cofilin. Its action is particularly effective in the absence of tropomyosin, which instead stabilizes the actin filaments. Cofilin preferentially binds to ADP-containing actin and thus tends to target the older microfilaments. As a consequence, it accelerates the actin filament turnover that is necessary during cell migration. Capping proteins stop microfilament elongation, avoiding extensive polymerization far from the plasma membrane. For recent review on actin-binding proteins, see reference 4.

Cell Migration

Cell migration onto solid surfaces comprises several steps, although the details vary between cell types and species.[5-8] On sensing external signals, cells undergo anteroposterior polarization, followed by extension of membrane protrusions at the front edge. These are generally rich in microfilaments and, depending on actin organization, can be divided in filopodia (meaning 'thread-like feets', subtle protrusions containing parallel actin bundles), lamellipodia ('laminar feets', flat expansions containing branched microfilaments) and pseudopodia ('pseudo-feets', finger-like extensions containing three-dimensional actin networks). During protrusion, the actin web undergoes polymerisation at the front and depolymerisation at the rear. Subsequently, the actin cytoskeleton at the migrating front attaches to the substratum through adhesion points. This is necessary to provide anchorage for the bulk of the cell to be drawn forward ('traction' phase). Traction forces are probably generated mainly by interaction of microfilaments with the bipolar myosin II, which allows the actin cortex contraction necessary to translocate the cell body and nucleus. In parallel, selective weakening of the adhesive contacts on the rear of the cell occurs, to bring about retraction of the trailing process (the final stage). It is thus clear that different regulatory processes must occur at the leading and at the trailing edge and that the balance of the adhesive and contracting structures regulates the overall rapidity of migration.[9]

The complex cytoskeletal rearrangements that accompany cell locomotion can be stimulated by diffusible chemicals, to produce random migration (chemokinesis) or directional migration (chemotaxis).[5] In addition, cell migration can be driven by cell-cell adhesion molecules or proteins of the extracellular matrix (ECM). Usually, long-distance migration depends on a combination of signals that coordinate the sequence of protrusion/adhesion/contraction/release steps along the cell's path. As typical mediators of cell interaction with the ECM, integrins play major roles in this process. Nonetheless, irrespective of the membrane receptor involved, most of the guidance signals are transduced into common intracellular regulatory pathways, in which a major role is exerted by the monomeric GTPase proteins of the Rho family (particularly Cdc42, Rac and RhoG). Rho stimulates microfilament bundle nucleation and polymerisation by activating the formins and inhibiting cofilamin. It also stimulates contraction by regulating myosin II, whose regulation is complex and also depends on cytosolic Ca^{2+} (see later). The ensuing promotion of stress fibers leads to integrin clustering and formation of adhesion plaques. Conversely, Rac (and/or Cdc42) stimulates the formation of actin networks through a complex regulatory cascade that inhibits myosin and activates the ARP complex (through the WASP/WAVE family of activators) and filamin. These regulatory mechanisms cooperate to produce well coordinated cytoskeletal dynamics, during cell crawling. Work carried out in neutrophils, fibroblasts, *Dictyostelium* and other cell types has provided a general background for chemotaxis.[7] When a membrane receptor binds a chemoattractant, local actin polimerization is stimulated. In particular, activation of phosphatidylinositol 3'-kinase (PI(3)K) produces phosphatidylinositol (3,4,5) trisphosphate (PIP_3). This latter activates Rac and thus ARP, with ensuing lamellipodial protrusion. PIP_3 is rapidly degraded to phosphatidylinositol (3,4) bisphosphate (PIP_2) by a lipid phosphatase. Therefore, a significant concentration of PIP_3 is only present at the front of the migrating cell. In parallel, chemoattractant binding also stimulates Rho and thus myosin, by a different mechanisms. Because these pathways inhibit each other, the overall result is that Rac activation prevails in the migrating front, whereas Rho prevails in the rear. In this way, a functional cellular polarity is maintained, so that protrusion occurs at the front and contraction at the rear.[1,7]

Growth Cone Motility

During development, neurons reach their final destination by exploiting the mechanisms outlined above. The subsequent formation of the highly branched neuronal shape also depends on actin cytoskeleton. Axon and dendrites' elongation continues until the appropriate synaptic contacts with target neurons are established. Both neuronal migration and neurite extension are led by ECM guidance signals and cell-cell adhesion molecules. The process does not cease after synaptic maturation, but continues throughout life and gives a major contribution to synaptic remodeling.[10,11] Recent results suggest that the growth cones may be the only part of the cell to be sensitive to the external guidance cues.[12] Considering how far from the cell body can growth cones travel, this observation suggests that in neurons the presence of sophisticated regulatory mechanisms capable of coordinating contraction and adhesion at distant cellular locations is particularly important. Nonetheless, the basic mechanisms of growth cone motility are thought to be broadly similar to those illustrated above and based on studies in non neuronal cells. The tips of axons and dendrites are rich in actin and emit filopodia and lamellipodia depending on environmental signals that stimulate the usual Rho-centered intracellular cascades.[13] Filopodia and lamellipodia form the so-called P(peripheral)-region, whereas the round-shape apex of the neurite shaft, from which those protrusions extend, is called C(central)-region. The C-region also contains microtubules and organelles. Growth cone advance depends on interaction between actin and microtubules. The initial actin-dependent protrusions are followed by advancement of the C-region, which is then stabilized as part of the neurite shaft. Once again, movement is guided by both fixed and diffusible signals, whose interplay produces exquisitely regulated movement. Growth cones can control the rate of advancement and pause, turn, or retract.[10] For instance, when growing neurites meet external signposts, they forms adhesion sites and then turn towards the signal. The mechanism is only partially understood and is probably driven by a myosin-dependent collapse of the actin network in the unstabilized part of the growth cone. In general, evidence suggests that Cdc42 and Rac control growth cone attraction, whereas RhoA is implicated in growth cone collapse and repulsion.[14,15] Both regulatory proteins and the contraction machinery are regulated by Ca^{2+} signals, as is further discussed later. When necessary, growing neurites can also bifurcate or fasciculate.

The Role of Integrins in Cell Migration

In many cell types, integrin receptors provide anchorage to the substratum and connect the adhesion sites to the contracting microfilaments. Connection between the adhesion and contraction machineries is necessary for efficient cell movement and is mediated by an array of adapter proteins. It should be recalled however that integrin-independent migration can occur in neurons (whose movement depends on a variety of extracellular signposts),[16] three-dimensional leukocyte chemotaxis[17] and tumor cells, in certain conditions.[18] Once engaged, integrins tend to cluster at adhesion sites, thus nucleating the assembly of structural and regulatory protein complexes (see Chapter 1). Adhesion points are linked to the actin cytoskeleton and stimulate migration-related intracellular factors.[8] Generally, active integrins tend to be located at the leading edge,[19] where they regulate the role of Rac/Cdc42 in protrusion.[20,21] The mechanism of adhesion site assembly is still matter of debate, but it is also thought to depend on Rac/Cdc42.[9] The more rapidly the cell migrates, the less evident integrin clusters are. Focal adhesion sites, with large integrin clusters, are typical of stationary or very slowly moving cells. As typical bidirectional signal transducers, integrins also control the strength of cell adhesion by changing the affinity of their extracellular domains for the substrate, in response to cytoplasmic signals that target the integrin cytoplasmic tail.[8]

Current evidence indicates that actin polymerization controls both the assembly and the structure of adhesion complexes at the leading front. Disassembled actin supports the maintenance of small adhesion points, whereas bundled actin sustains large elongated adhesion sites, which tend to assemble along the actin filaments. Once again, a bidirectional relation seems to take place between actin cytoskeleton and adhesion sites. Actin polymerization determines the rate of assembly of adhesion complexes, by associating with integrins at the leading edge and controlling their positioning at the tip of the microfilament.[22,23] Conversely, integrin complexes may provide nucleating sites for polymerizing actin.[24] For review of this rapidly growing field, see ref. 8. Many aspects of the interplay between the integrin-centered multiprotein complexes and the cytoskeleton are mediated by Rho proteins, with the important contribution of paxillin, a 'hub' which connects the elements of these complex structures. In addition, posttranslational modifications of the cytoplasmic domains can control integrin affinity during migration. For example, phosphorylation of $\alpha 4$ integrin at the leading process leads to paxillin release. The ensuing lamellipodium stabilization serves for cells to migrate on α4β1-adhesive ECM.[25] For efficient retraction of the trailing edge and emission of new protrusions at the leading edge, controlled disassembly of adhesion sites is also necessary. Adhesion turnover seems to be under the control of microtubule dynamics and pathways involving the focal adhesion kinase (FAK), the extracellular signal regulated kinase (ERK) and Src, at both the anterior an posterior sides. A full picture is still unavailable,[8,9] nonetheless the contribution of Ca^{2+} signals at the rear side is probably crucial. It has been suggested that strong traction activates stretch-activated Ca^{2+} channels.[26] Ca^{2+} influx may activate the phosphatase calcineurin and the protease calpain. The latter, besides being also regulated by ERK, is known to cleave proteins of the adhesion machinery, such as integrin subunits, talin, vinculin and FAK.[27] Finally, retraction at the rear edge depends on myosin, which is controlled by a Rho-dependent cascade.[9]

The Role of Ion Channels and Crosstalk with Integrins in Cell Migration

The literature on ion channels and cell motility is steadily increasing. In the following paragraphs, with no pretension of exhaustiveness, we illustrate a few examples that are selected to convey (i) a general notion of the main physiological issues and their pathological implications and (ii) information about current trends in the field.

K+ Channels

It is now recognized that Ca^{2+}-activated and voltage-dependent K+ channels are implicated in cell movement regulation. K+ channel activation tends to produce membrane hyperpolarization (see Chapter 2) and thus increases the electrochemical gradient for Ca^{2+}. The ensuing Ca^{2+} influx has manifold effects on cell migration.[10,28] Moreover, migration is accompanied by cell shape rearrangements that require local volume alteration. In general, the transmembrane water fluxes that occur during regulated cell volume changes are driven by osmotic forces that depend on modification of the intracellular concentration of NaCl, KCl and organic compounds such as certain aminoacids, taurin and others. The details are different between cell types and species. Nevertheless, a common mechanism to bring about regulatory volume decrease on cell swelling involves KCl efflux caused by coordinated activation of K+ and Cl- channels, at least in the early phases of the process. A comprehensive review on mammalian cell volume regulation is ref. 29. K+ and Cl- channels cooperate in controlling cell volume alterations in both normal and neoplastic cells.[30,31] These processes are particularly relevant from our standpoint since cell volume is known to regulate the actin cytoskeleton.[32] This as well as other lines of evidence show that cell volume control is strictly linked to cell adhesion and migration.[29]

Besides volume control, several K+ channel types are implicated in regulating the migration machinery in other ways. They can form molecular complexes with cortactin,[33,34] FAK[35,36] and integrin subunits.[37] Alternatively, such a coupling may be mediated by intracellular messengers.[37] In the following, we examine some detailed studies focused on the α4β1 and α9β1 integrins. Although most integrin types regulate migration, α4β1 and α9β1 are functionally related in that they tend to produce simultaneous stimulation of cell movement and inhibition of spreading. However, the mechanisms involved are different.[38] In T-lymphocytes, a classical model for studying cell migration, phosphorylation of the α4β1 integrin expressed at the leading edge increases lamellipodial protrusion, whereas retraction at the trailing edge is facilitated by dephosphorylation. This process is mediated by Rac, which is activated when paxillin binds to the integrin C-terminus.[9,25,39-41] Although the α9-containing integrins also bind paxillin,[39,42] recent results suggest that they regulate cell movement by activating inward rectifier K+ channels (IRK).[43] As is discussed in Chapter 2, open IRK channels allow much larger currents when K+ is flowing inward, i.e., when the membrane potential is more negative than the K+ equilibrium potential. This property (inward rectification) is caused by the voltage-dependent channel block produced by intracellular organic cations (and Mg^{2+}) that tend to occlude the channel pore when ions flow from the intracellular to the extracellular space. The main organic cations producing this effect are spermine and spermidine, polyamines normally present in the cytoplasm of most mammalian cells.

That polyamines are implicated in cell movement regulation was suggested by studies showing that the migration of intestinal epithelial cells depends on polyamines, probably through activation of Rac1.[44] Subsequent work carried out in Chinese hamster ovary cells pointed out that binding of the spermidine/spermine N[1]-acetyltransferase to the cytoplasmic domain of α9 integrin is sufficient to stimulate cell migration.[45] This enzyme catalyzes the rate limiting step along the pathway that acetylates spermine (valence +4) and spermidine (+3) to putrescine (+2). Because of lower charge, acetylated polyamines are much less effective in channel inhibition. Moreover, they are more efficiently extruded or metabolized by the cell, which further lowers their potency as IRK blockers.[46] More recent results from D. Sheppard's research laboratory show that functional spermidine/spermine N[1]-acetyltransferase and an adequate intracellular concentration of these polyamines are necessary for proper α9β1-dependent cell movement. As expected, the effect depends precisely on modulation of an IRK-type channel, namely Kir4.2. Blocking either the activity or the expression of Kir4.2 in engineered cell lines and microvascular endothelial cells inhibits the α9 dependent cell migration. In fact, Kir4.2 colocalizes with α9β1 integrin in focal adhesion complexes, at the front of the crawling cells.[43] This work thus provides another way through which integrins and ion channels can communicate. The importance for cell crawling control seems established, although the specific role of IRK channels in migration is still unclear.

Nicotinic Acetylcholine Receptors, Integrins and Epithelial Migration in Electric Fields, Implications for Wound Healing

The 'neuronal' nicotinic acetylcholine receptors (nAChRs) are widely expressed in non neuronal tissues as well.[47] In these, cholinergic agonists can stimulate chemotaxis by activating nAChRs.[47,48] This process has been thoroughly studied in epithelial keratinocytes, in which stimulation of nAChRs by paracrine release of ACh controls the cell locomotion necessary to bring about epithelial renewal and wound healing. Steady electric fields perpendicular to the wound axis are known to be present in epithelia, including the mammalian skin.[49] Keratinocytes tend to migrate along the field lines (a process named galvanotropism), to repair the wound.[50] When cells migrate in the presence of an electric field, several types of ion channels cluster at the leading front.[51,52] In migrating human keratinocytes, in particular, the α7 nAChR subunit clusters at the leading edge and colocalizes with the β1 integrin. Interestingly, a metabotropic ACh receptor, the M1 muscarinic receptor, also clusters at the leading edge. Specific inhibition of either homomeric α7 nAChRs or M1 muscarinic receptors blocks the chemotaxis occurring along gradients of cholinergic agonists. On the other hand, random keratinocyte chemokinesis seems to be under prevalent control of heteromeric nAChR receptors. The α7 nAChRs are highly permeable to Ca^{2+}. As was briefly mentioned in Chapter 9, activation of M1 receptors and α7 nAChRs cooperate in stimulating intracellular cascades that converge onto the Ras/Raf/MEK1/ERK pathway. In more detail, activation of the Raf/MEK/ERK cascade is activated by a combination of a Ca^{2+}-independent (mediated by Ras) and a Ca^{2+} dependent pathway (through the Ca^{2+}-calmodulin dependent protein kinase II and protein kinase C).[48,53,54] The relation with integrin physiology depends on the fact that activation of the above pathway up-regulates the α2 and α3 integrins, which have the usual function of stabilizing the lamellipodia.

Interesting parallel work on the cytoskeletal reorganization that accompanies keratinocyte migration in the presence of electric fields points to the activation of PI(3)Kγ and the tumor suppressor phosphatase and tensin homolog (PTEN).[55] To provide a link between the electrical fields across epithelial wounds and such intracellular responses, these authors provided evidence of the involvement of the Na^+/H^+ exchanger 1 (NHE1) and Cl^- channels.[55] Is there also evidence of a functional link between nAChRs and the above regulatory pathways? Recent work suggests that there is, because activating nAChRs in keratinocytes leads to stimulate Jak2 phosphorylation, which is connected to the PI(3)K/ROK cascade that regulates microfilament reorganization.[54]

Ca²⁺ Signaling and the Axonal Growth Cone

Largely common Ca²⁺-dependent signaling pathways regulate neuronal migration, neurite extension and synaptic remodeling. In particular, similar mechanisms of growth cone guidance take place both at the axonal and the dendritic tips. Typically, extracellular cues trigger Ca²⁺ influx through membrane channels, such as voltage-gated Ca²⁺ channels, Ca²⁺-permeable ligand-gated channels and transient receptor potential (TRP) channels.[10,56] We first briefly review the fundamentals of intracellular Ca²⁺ signaling and its role in cell movement. Next, we illustrate what is known about growth cone motility, which provides a clear example of the complexity of Ca²⁺ signals in cell migration.

Ca²⁺ Signals: Fundamentals and Role in Chemotaxis

Because of the Ca²⁺ buffering capacity of many cytosolic proteins, this ion diffuses very slowly in the cytoplasm.[57-59] As a consequence, Ca²⁺ influx tends to have local signaling roles around the entry site. To generate global increase of cytoplasmic Ca²⁺, the local signal must be amplified by massive Ca²⁺ release from the intracellular stores. Such a release is mediated by several channel types expressed in the membranes of the endoplasmic/sarcoplasmic reticulum, such as the ryanodine receptors (RyRs) and the inositol 1,4,5-trisphosphate receptors (IP₃Rs). RyRs and IP₃Rs comprise several subtypes and are sensitive to both Ca²⁺ and second messengers. The expression of these (and probably other) intracellular receptors varies in different cells. The interplay between RyRs and IP₃Rs (when they are coexpressed) is only beginning to be understood. For examples in sea urchin embryos and mammalian neurons see refs. 60-61, respectively. In resting conditions, the cytosolic [Ca²⁺] is maintained around 100 nM by Ca²⁺ ATPases located at both the plasma membrane and the membranes of internal stores and by the Na⁺/Ca²⁺ exchanger. During stimulation, free intracellular Ca²⁺ can rise to micromolar levels.[10,62] Depleted intracellular stores can be refilled by extracellular Ca²⁺ influx through specific membrane channels operated by intracellular stores, a process named capacitive Ca²⁺ entry.[63] The main components of the cellular apparatus that controls Ca²⁺ homeostasis are illustrated in Figure 1.

The dynamics of intracellular Ca²⁺ can be determined by using the fluorescent Ca²⁺ indicators originally based on the structure of EGTA[64] or, more recently, by detecting the Förster resonance energy transfer (FRET, see Chapter 4) signal produced by the conformational change occurring on Ca²⁺ binding to calmodulin.[65] The history of the studies about the role of Ca²⁺ signals in neuronal migration and neurite extension is found in ref. 10. Work in immune cells,[66,67] epithelial keratinocytes[29] and cerebellar neurons[68] suggests that often a stable rear-to-front Ca²⁺ gradient is formed in cells during chemotaxis, which is thought to be one of the causes of the different behavior of the front and rear side, with retraction and detachment of the trailing edge during the the last phase of the cell movement cycle. In other experimental systems, transient Ca²⁺ increases at the cell front have been implicated in protrusion of the leading edge.[69] Therefore, transient Ca²⁺ signals probably stimulate the cytoskeleton, whereas steady signals control the anteroposterior polarity. Therefore, the more efficient pattern of Ca²⁺ stimulation seems to be different for the cytoskeleton and the apparatus that senses directional signals. Another example is provided by experiments carried out in cerebellar granule cells. When these are challenged with Slit-2 (a neuronal repellent, i.e., a directional signal), they produce a Ca²⁺ wave that propagates from the growth cone to the neuronal soma.[12]

Growth Cone Motility

Growth cone extension requires a permissive range of $[Ca^{2+}]_i$,[70] whereas the frequency of Ca²⁺ waves and spikes controls the rate of axonal elongation.[71] More localized Ca²⁺ transients produce asymmetrical cone movements that are responsible for cone steering in response to extracellular guidance signals.[71-74] The effects of Ca²⁺ depend on regulation of the cytoskeletal dynamics, which is mediated by a vast array of intracellular Ca²⁺-sensitive molecular targets. The most obvious is myosin, which is stimulated when the myosin light chain kinase (MLCK) is activated by association with the Ca²⁺/calmodulin (CaM) complex. This mechanism indeed regulates growth cone motility.[75] However, there is much more to the effects of intracellular Ca²⁺ on cell motility.

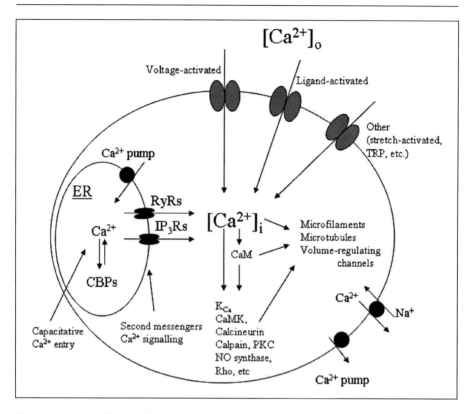

Figure 1. Ca^{2+} signaling and homeostasis in mammalian cells. Schema of the main processes implicated in the regulation of intracellular Ca^{2+} concentration ($[Ca^{2+}]_i$) and list of some cellular targets of Ca^{2+} described in the main text. $[Ca^{2+}]_o$: extracellular Ca^{2+} concentration; CBP: Ca^{2+} binding proteins (like calsequestrin or calretinin) that buffer Ca^{2+} within the endoplasmic/sarcoplasmic reticulum; CaMK: Ca^{2+}-calmodulin dependent protein kinase; ER: endoplasmic reticulum; IP_3R: receptor for IP_3; K_{Ca}: Ca^{2+}-activated K^+ channels; PKC: protein kinase C (i.e., Ca^{2+} dependent); RyR: ryanodine receptor; TRP: transient receptor potential channels.

For detailed review, see ref. 10. We briefly mention that the cytoskeletal and neurite dynamics is thought to be modulated through different forms of CaM-dependent kinases (CaMK)[74,76,77] and Ca^{2+} dependent phosphatases like calcineurin.[78] Moreover, the Ca^{2+}-CaM complex is also known to regulate the nitric oxide (NO) synthase, both directly and through the mediation of CaMKII and calcineurin.[79] The level of NO regulates the cGMP-dependent protein kinases, which are also involved in neurite extension and neuronal migration.[10] As previously discussed, the Rho GTPases are major regulators of cell motility. Rho proteins are under control of GTPase activating proteins (GAPs) and guanine nucleotide exchange factors (GEFs), both of which appear to be regulated by cytoplasmic Ca^{2+}.[80] In addition, Rho GTPases are also controlled by protein kinase C and CaMKII.[81,82] Many other proteins implicated in the dynamics of actin cytoskeleton are thought to be regulated by Ca^{2+}, such as gelsolin, ROCK and others. Finally, the microtubule associated proteins are also targets of Ca^{2+} signaling.[10]

The coordination of adhesion points' turnover, i.e., assembly at the front and disassembly at the rear of moving cells, is particularly delicate in the long neuronal processes. Further complexity is added by the variety of fixed adhesion cues present in the developing nervous system, including ECM, radial glia and the surfaces of surrounding neurons. Knowledge about these processes is far from being complete, although one can assume that the mechanisms determined in other experimental systems should broadly apply to the nervous system as well. In particular, Rho GTPases are implicated in regulating the adhesion contacts formed by growth cones.[83] It is thus conceivable that the Ca^{2+} signals discussed above may also control the dynamics of neurite adhesion to the substrate. Disassembly is instead controlled by the microtubule dynamics[84] and work in fibroblasts suggests that this is mainly regulated by dynamin and FAK and not Rho.[85] It has been proposed that the role of Ca^{2+} could be the regulation of disassembly, through control of endocytosis.[10] The hypothesis is based on the observation that clathrin-mediated endocytosis of β1 integrins occurs in migrating cells, when cell motility is stimulated by inducing clustering of the cell-adhesion protein L1, in HEK293 cells.[86]

In analogy with what has been observed in other cell types,[37] in growth cones the adhesion machinery could feed-back and regulate Ca^{2+} signaling. No evidence is still available for integrins, but the cell adhesion molecules (CAMs) expressed on cultured dorsal root ganglion neurons can steer growth cones by local stimulation of the RyR Type 3.[87] The link between the pattern of neuronal activity and the expression of membrane receptors that respond to fixed or diffusible guidance cues is still largely unexplored. Nonetheless, we predict interesting future developments on the basis of (i) growing evidence along similar lines in non neuronal cells;[37] (ii) the relation between glutamate ionotropic receptor activity and integrin expression in hippocampal cells (see Chapter 9) and (iii) several observations showing that the expression of CAMs changes depending on the pattern of neuronal discharge.[88,89]

Ion Channels as Adhesion Molecules

The relation between the extracellular environment and ion channels is not always mediated by membrane receptors such as integrins or CAMs. In neuromuscular junction preparations, the presynaptic voltage-gated Ca^{2+} channels have been shown to directly bind to laminin β2.[90] Such an interaction takes place also when sensory neurons grow on appropriate surfaces. N. Spitzer and colleagues[91] have studied the stop signal that serves to induce sensory axons to cease growing when they arrive in the skin. When the growing axons of spinal *Xenopus* neurons encounter a surface coated with laminin β2, they produce intracellular Ca^{2+} transients and pause. Ca^{2+} influx is necessary for the growth cones to stop moving and depends, at least, on voltage-gated calcium channels (Ca$_V$2.2)[91] and on mechanosensitive channels[92] expressed onto the growth cone membrane. The stop signal is however not mediated by integrin receptors, but in all probability by laminin forming a complex with the Ca$_V$2.2 channel itself.[91] A further example concerns voltage-gated Na$^+$ channels. The accessory β1 subunit behaves both as a cell-cell and cell-matrix adhesion protein, depending on context. It can thus affect neurite outgrowth and neuronal development in general. A concise introduction to literature is found in ref. 93. This role of voltage-gated Na$^+$ channels is suggestive also in the light of the evidence showing that they are implicated in late stages of neoplasia. For instance, the Na$_V$1.7 channel is associated with strong metastatic potential in prostate cancer in vitro and its activity potentiates cell migration.[94,95] These intriguing, although still fragmentary, evidences bring us to consider the possible implications of the processes outlined in the previous paragraphs for the metastatic process.

The Cellular Environment and the Metastatic Process

Recent studies have led to ample revision of the traditional view of cancer as a disease caused by groups of transformed cells acquiring cell autonomous hyperproliferative, invasive and limitless survival capacities. Current views point out that carcinogenesis and tumor progression need to be considered not so much as conditions centered on largely autonomous cancer cells, but rather as complex disease processes involving heterotypic multicellular interactions within a newly formed tissue, the cancer tissue. This notion has led to the concept of tumor microenvironment (TM), as an integrated and essential part of the cancer tissue.[96] According to this view, the therapeutic strategies that have been so far concentrated on targeting the tumor cell itself are better turned to target the tumor as well as the TM as a whole. Thus, from both a theoretical and a practical viewpoint, knowledge and control of the TM is becoming as important as knowledge and control of the neoplastic cell.

The TM surrounding the malignant cells, also called the "tumor stroma", consists of the non malignant cells as well as the tumor ECM, which contains, among the other components, a multitude of growth factors that affect tumor growth. The tumor stroma contains many distinct cell types, including endothelial cells and their precursors, pericytes, smooth muscle cells, fibroblasts, carcinoma-associated fibroblasts, myofibroblasts, neutrophils, eosinophils, basophils, T- and B- lymphocytes, natural killer cells, macrophages and dendritic cells.[97] Although the stromal cells are not malignant in that they do not bear cancerogenic mutations, they do exhibit epigenetic changes, which affect their behavior and protein expression. Nevertheless, the ECM-producing cells inside the TM are generally activated and this leads to a defensive mechanism known as tumor desmoplasia. The desmoplastic reaction tends to confine the tumor and prevents further neoplastic growth. It is thought to be an active process, which participates in several aspects of tumor progression such as angiogenesis, invasion and metastasis. Moreover, current evidence suggests that tumor desmoplasia is the main determinant of tumor chemoresistance.[98]

The reactive stroma of a tumor presents high vascularity, is associated with numerous ECM-producing fibroblasts and shows increased production of ECM products such as collagens. The cancer cells and stroma both modulate their ECM by secreting cancer-associated proteases, which attack proteins like collagens, proteoglycans, etc. This remodeling process leads to the release of molecules sequestered in the ECM, such as the vascular endothelial growth factor (VEGF)[99] and many cleavage products of ECM proteins.[96,100,101] These molecules further control the neoplastic progression. In particular, normal epithelia are always associated with a basement membrane (BM), a highly specialized ECM containing many proteins, among which we remind Type IV collagen, laminin, Types XV and XVIII collagens, perlecan and nidogen. As mentioned above, many of these proteins as well as domains cleaved from them can affect tumor progression. The cleaved fragments of BM proteins suppress tumor growth by inhibiting angiogenesis.[102] By definition, a tumor becomes invasive when it acquires the ability of penetrating the BM and infiltrating through the underlying normal stromal zone. Prior to BM invasion, the tumor is referred to as an in situ carcinoma. However, well before the BM is disrupted by cancer cells, these latter influence and activate the stroma. Typically, activation of stromal cells such as fibroblasts is observed within in situ carcinoma. The cooperation of proteases expressed by cancer cells and stroma cells tends to break down the BM barrier. In this way, both neoplastic and activated stromal cells affect tumor progression.[98]

Although it is the systemic metastatic spread of cancer that leads to the death of most cancer patients, the process of metastasis has traditionally received a lesser attention in cancer research. Since Paget's 'soil and seed' hypothesis, it has been evident that the development of metastases from a primary tumor is not a random process simply explained by the pattern of circulation.[103] The metastatic process requires many distinct steps such as loss of cell adhesion, increased motility and invasiveness, intravasation and survival in the blood stream, extravasation into the future site of metastasis and finally colonization of the distant sites that present a permissive soil.[104] A schema of the metastatic process is outlined in Figure 2. Once the malignant cells encounter the normal tissue stroma at the site of metastasis, it is vital for them to make this stroma permissive for the subsequent organization of the metastasis. Not much is known about the relative contribution to this process of the cancer cell itself, the cells within the stromal compartment of the primary tumor and the activating stems cells from the bone marrow. However, recent findings indicate that the role of mesenchymal stem cells is particularly relevant to confer increased metastatic potential to neoplastic cells. It is thus believed that the organization of metastasis is a dual process, in which the formation of a premetastatic niche facilitates the initial survival of metastatic cells. Subsequently, up-regulation occurs of the genes necessary to effectively colonize the new site. Not all seeded cells will develop into metastases. In fact, in many cancer types, tumor cells can be found in locations such as the bone marrow years before the development of a metastasis. Such a pattern also suggests that the cancer cell itself may require the development of metastasis to proceed along the

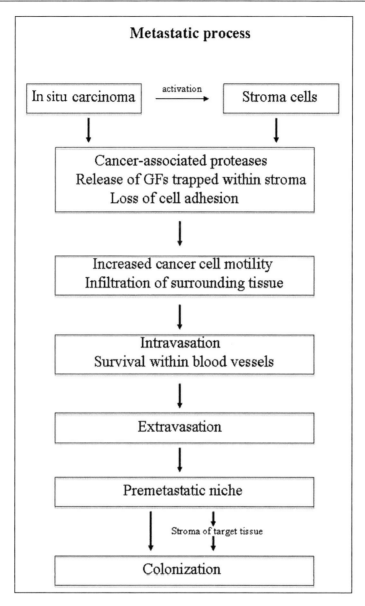

Figure 2. Schematic summary of the main steps in the metastatic process. The principal metastatic steps discussed in the text are summarized for reference. GF: growth factors. Intravasation: process of invasion of blood vessels by neoplastic cells migrating from the primary tumor site. Extravasation: invasion of target tissue by neoplastic cells circulating in blood.

malignant pathway and that the metastatic phenotype most likely depends on continuing interaction between tumor cells and stroma.[104]

Considering the importance of cell interaction with its environment and the control of cell adhesion and migration during the metastatic process, it is likely that future work will reveal an intricate regulatory network involving adhesion receptors and ion channels. Until now, however, specific examples exist concerning single aspects of the metastatic cascade. One of the best known examples is the function of ion channels in glioma cell migration, which we review in the following paragraph.

Invasiveness of Glial Tumors and Ion Channels

Glial tumors (gliomas) are the most common primary brain tumors and are broadly subdivided in astrocytomas, oligodendrogliomas, mixed oligoastrocytomas and ependimomas.[105] The malignant astrocytomas are the most aggressive and despite recent advances in chemotherapy, their prognosis remains poor.[106,107] A major reason for this severity is that glial tumors, instead of spreading through blood to produce distant metastases, are very effective in infiltrating the parenchyma of brain and spinal cord, thus potently colonizing their tissue of origin. This feature is particularly detrimental to surgical therapy.[107] Moreover, infiltrating glioma cells tend to decrease their proliferation rate and develop resistance to apoptosis compared to the tumor core, which is probably the reason for their unusual resistance to common therapy. Better results have been recently obtained by use of the chemotherapeutic compound temozolomide, which may partly circumvent the apoptotic resistance.[106,108] An alternative strategy for treatment is suggested by the observation that inhibiting the migration of actively moving glioma cells increases their sensitivity to proapoptotic compounds.[109,110] To move through the narrow interstitia, glioma cells need to achieve sophisticated control of their motility, shape and volume. Normal glial cells express a variety of voltage- and ligand-gated ion channels and aquaporins, whose role is still debated.[111-114] During development, proliferating glial cells express several voltage-gated K$^+$ channels and are relatively depolarized, whereas mature noncycling astrocytes have resting potentials around -80 mV, because of expression of IRK-type channels.[115-118] The balance of expression of voltage-gated and IRK K$^+$ channels in both astrocytes and oligodendrocytes is thought to be related to the cell cycle control.[119,120]

In glioma cell lines and primary samples, the cell shrinkage necessary for these cells to infiltrate through the narrow extracellular spaces of the central nervous system depends on KCl efflux brought about by activation of Cl$^-$ and K$^+$ channels, with water following osmotically through aquaporins.[31,121,122] The main K$^+$ channel expressed by gliomas is a high-conductance Ca^{2+}-activated channel (gBK), encoded by a splice variant of *KCNMA1* (or K_{Ca} *1.1*). A major physiological stimulus, in this context, is probably Ca^{2+} influx through Ca^{2+} permeable alpha-amino-3-hydroxy--5-methyl-4-isoxazolepropionic acid (AMPA) receptors, although gBK is also regulated by growth factors and neurotransmitters.[122] The Cl$^-$ current depends on activation of ClC-3, a channel typically found in endocytic vescicles.[121] Different inhibitors of these channels block glioma cell invasion. Interestingly, human glioma cells also express an amiloride-sensitive Na$^+$ current that is not found in normal astrocytes.[123] It is known that an important component of regulatory volume increase is influx of NaCl.[29] Therefore, activation of this current type may contribute to restoring cell volume after shrinking during migration within the cerebral interstice, or may contribute to the volume changes that accompany the cell cycle. Finally, overexpression of hERG voltage-gated K$^+$ channels has been observed in surgical samples from high-grade gliomas. Further work in glioma cell lines suggests that the hERG channel expression is not related to the volume control, but is implicated in the control of VEGF secretion.[124]

Conclusion

Ion transporters have been also implicated in the biology of gliomas. The best example is probably the Na$^+$/K$^+$ ATPase, whose α1 subunit is overexpressed in a fraction of glioblastomas.[110] In experimental models, it has been possible to decrease glioblastoma cell proliferation and migration by using highly specific sodium pump inhibitors. Treatment leads to microfilament disassembly, which is the likely cause of migration impairment and cell autophagy.[110] It is thus clear that the study of the implications of ion fluxes and transport proteins in the biology of metastasis is a complex and promising research field that we believe will lead to surprises from both a theoretical and a pharmacological point of view.

Acknowledgements

The authors' work is supported by the Italian Ministry for University and Scientific Research (PRIN), Associazione Genitori contro le Leucemie e Tumori Infantili Noi per Voi, Associazione Italiana per la Ricerca sul Cancro, Istituto Toscano Tumori, Ente Cassa di Risparmio di Firenze, Fondazione Città della Speranza, University of Milano Bicocca (FAR).

References

1. Alberts B, Johnson A, Lewis J et al. Molecular Biology of the Cell, 5th ed. Garland Science, 2008.
2. Bray D. Cell Movements: From Molecules to Motility, 2nd ed. Garland Science, 2001.
3. Zigmond SH. Formin-induced nucleation of actin filaments. Curr Opin Cell Biol 2004; 16:99-105.
4. dos Remedios CG, Chhabra D, Kekic M et al. Actin binding proteins: regulation of cytoskeletal microfilaments. Physiol Rev 2003; 83:433-473.
5. Lauffenburger DA, Horwitz AF. Cell migration, a physically integrated molecular process. Cell 1996; 84:359-369.
6. Le Clainche C, Carlier MF. Regulation of actin assembly associated with protrusion and adhesion in cell migration. Physiol Rev 2008; 88:489-513.
7. Wiener OD. Regulation of cell polarity during eukaryotic chemotaxis: the chemotactic compass. Curr Opin Cell Biol 2002; 14:196-202.
8. Vicente-Manzanares M, Choi CK, Horwitz AR. Integrins in cell migration—the actin connection. J Cell Sci 2009; 122:199-206.
9. Ridley AJ, Schwartz MA, Burridge K et al. Cell migration: integrating signals from front to back. Science 2003; 302:1704-1709.
10. Zheng JQ, Poo MM. Calcium signaling in neuronal motility. Annu Rev Cell Dev Biol 2007; 23:375-404.
11. Ayala R, Shu T, Tsai LH. Trekking across the brain: the journey of neuronal migration. Cell 2007; 128:29-43.
12. Guan CB, Xu HT, Jin M et al. Long-range Ca^{2+} signaling from growth cone to soma mediates reversal of neuronal migration induced by Slit-2. Cell 2007; 129:385-395.
13. Fukata M, Nakagawa M, Kaibuchi K. Roles of Rho-family GTPases in cell polarisation and directional migration. Curr Opin Cell Biol 2003; 15:590-597.
14. Dickson BJ. Rho GTPases in growth cone guidance. Curr Opin Neurobiol 2001; 11:103-110.
15. Yuan XB, Jin M, Xu C et al. Signaling and crosstalk of Rho GTPases in mediating axon guidance. Nat Cell Biol 2003; 5:38-45.
16. Maness PF, Schachner M. Neural recognition molecules of the immunoglobulin superfamily: signaling transducers of axon guidance and neuronal migration. Nat Neurosci 2007; 10:19-26.
17. Lammermann T, Bader BL, Monkley SJ et al. Rapid leukocyte migration by integrin-independent flowing and squeezing. Nature 2008; 453:51-55.
18. Wolf K, Wu YI, Liu Y et al. Multi-step pericellular proteolysis controls the transition from individual to collective cancer cell invasion. Nat Cell Biol 9:893-904.
19. Kiosses WB, Shattil SJ, Pampori N et al. Rac recruits high-affinity integrin alphaVbeta3 to lamellipodia in endothelial cell migration. Nat Cell Biol 2001; 3:316-320.
20. Kraynov VS, Chamberlain C, Bokoch GM et al. Localized Rac activation dynamics visualized in living cells. Science 2000; 290:333-337.
21. Nalbant P, Hodgson L, Kraynov V et al. Activation of endogenous Cdc42 visualized in living cells. Science 2004; 305:1615-1619.
22. Galbraith CG, Yamada KM, Galbraith JA. Polymerizing actin fibers position integrins primed to probe for adhesion sites. Science 2007; 315:992-995.
23. Choi CK, Vicente-Manzanares M, Zareno J. Actin and alpha-actinin orchestrate the assembly and maturation of nascent adhesions in a myosin II motor-independent manner. Nat Cell Biol 2008; 10:1039-1050.
24. Butler B, Gao C, Mersich AT et al. Purified integrin adhesion complexes exhibit actin-polymerization activity. Curr Biol 2006; 16:242-251.
25. Goldfinger LE, Han J, Kiosses WB et al. Spatial restriction of alpha4 integrin phosphorylation regulates lamellipodial stability and alpha4beta1 dependent cell migration. J Cell Biol 2003; 162:731-741.
26. Lee J, Ishihara A, Oxford G et al. Regulation of cell movement is mediated by stretch-activated calcium channels. Nature 1999; 400:382-386.
27. Glading A, Lauffenburger DA, Wells A. Cutting to the chase: calpain proteases in cell motility. Trends Cell Biol 2002; 12:46-54.
28. Schwab A, Hanley P, Fabian A et al. Potassium channels keep mobile cells on the go. Physiology 2008; 23:212-220.

29. Hoffmann EK, Lambert IH, Pedersen SF. Physiology of cell volume regulation in vertebrates. Physiol Rev 2009; 89:193-277.
30. Schwab A, Nechyporuk-Zloy V, Fabian A et al. Cells move when ions and water flow. Pflugers Arch 2007; 453:421-432.
31. Sontheimer H. An unexpected role for ion channels in brain tumor metastasis. Exp Biol Med 2008; 233:779-791.
32. Pedersen SF, Hoffmann EK, Mills JW. The cytoskeleton and cell volume regulation. Comp Biochem Physiol A 2001; 130:385-399.
33. Tian L, Chen L, McClafferty H et al. A noncanonical SH3 domain binding motif links BK channels to the actin cytoskeleton via the SH3 adapter cortactin. FASEB J 2006; 20:2588-2590.
34. Williams MR, Markey JC, Doczi MA et al. An essential role for cortactin in the modulation of the potassium channel Kv1.2. Proc Natl Acad Sci USA 2007; 104:17412-17417.
35. Rezzonico R, Cayatte C, Bourget-Ponzio I et al. Focal adhesion kinase pp125FAK interacts with the large conductance calcium-activated hSlo potassium channel in human osteoblasts: potential role in mechanotransduction. J Bone Miner Res 2003; 18:1863-1871.
36. Wei J-F, Wei L, Zhou X et al. Formation of Kv2.1-FAK complex as a mechanism of FAK activation, cell polarization and enhanced motility. J Cell Physiol 2008; 217:544-557.
37. Arcangeli A, Becchetti A. Complex functional interaction between integrin receptors and ion channels. Trends Cell Biol 2006; 16:631-639.
38. Vandenberg CA. Integrins step up the pace of cell migration through polyamines and potassium channels. Proc Natl Acad Sci (USA) 2008; 105:7109-7110.
39. Liu S, Slepak M, Ginsberg MH. Binding of paxillin to the $\alpha 9$ integrin cytoplasmic domain inhibits cell spreading. J Biol Chem 2001; 276:37086-37092.
40. Han J, Rose DM, Woodside DG et al. Integrin alpha 4 beta 1-dependent T-cell migration requires both phosphorylation and dephosphorylation of the alpha 4 cytoplasmic domain to regulate the reversible binding of paxillin. J Biol Chem 2003; 278:34845-34853.
41. Rose DM, Alon R, Ginsberg MH. Integrin modulation and signaling in leukocyte adhesion and migration. Immunol Rev 2007; 218:126-134.
42. Young BA, Taooka Y, Liu S et al. The cytoplasmic domain of the integrin $\alpha 9$ subunit requires the adaptor protein paxillin to inhibit cell spreading but promotes cell migration in a paxillin-independent manner. Mol Biol Cell 2001; 12:3214-3225.
43. deHart G-W, Jin T, McCloskey DE et al. The $\alpha 9\beta 1$ integrin enhances cell migration by polyamine-mediated modulation of an inward-rectifier potassium channel. Proc Natl Acad Sci (USA) 2008; 105:7188-7193.
44. Ray RM, McCormack SA, Covington C et al. The requirement for polyamines for intestinal epithelial cell migration is mediated through Rac1. J Biol Chem 2003; 278:13039-13046.
45. Chen C, Young BA, Coleman CS et al. Spermidine/spermine N1-acetyltransferase specifically binds to the integrin $\alpha 9$ subunit cytoplasmic domain and enhances cell migration. J Cell Biol 2004; 167:161-170.
46. Pegg AE. Spermidine/spermine-N(1)-acetyltransferase: a key metabolic regulator. Am J Physiol Endocrinol Metab 2008; 294:E995-E1010.
47. Wessler I, Kirkpatrick CJ. Acetylcholine beyond neurons: the nonneuronal cholinergic system in humans. Br J Pharmacol 2008; 154:1558-1571.
48. Chernyavsky AI, Arredondo J, Marubio LM et al. Differential regulation of keratinocyte chemokinesis and chemotaxis through distinct nicotinic receptors subtypes. J Cell Sci 2004; 117:5665-5679.
49. McCaig CD, Raynicek AM, Song B et al. Controlling cell behaviour electrically: current views and future potential. Physiol Rev 2005; 85:943-978.
50. Nishimura KY, Isseroff RR, Nuccitelli R. Human keratinocytes migrate to the negative pole in direct current electric fields comparable to those measured in mammalian wounds. J Cell Sci 1996; 109:199-207.
51. Luther PW, Peng HB. Membrane-related specializations associated with acetylcholine receptor aggregates induced by electric fields. J Cell Biol 1985; 100:235-244.
52. Peng HB, Baker LP, Dai Z. A role of tyrosine phosphorylation in the formation of acetylcholine receptor clusters induced by electric fields in cultured Xenopus muscle cells. J Cell Biol 1993; 120:197-204.
53. Chernyavsky AI, Arredondo J, Karlsson E et al. The Ras/Raf-1/MEK1/ERK signaling pathway coupled to integrin expression mediates cholinergic regulation of keratinocyte directional migration. J Biol Chem 2005; 280:39220-39228.
54. Chernyavsky AI, Arredondo J, Qian J et al. Coupling of ionic events to protein kinase signaling cascades upon activation of $\alpha 7$ nicotinic receptor. Cooperative regulation of α_2-integrin expression and Rho-kinase activity. J Biol Chem 2009; 284:22140-22148.
55. Zhao M, Song B, Pu J et al. Electric signals control wound healing through phosphatidylinositol-3-OH kinase-γ and PTEN. Nature 2006; 442:457-460.

56. Spitzer NC. Electrical activity in early neuronal development. Nature 2006; 444:707-712.
57. Albritton NL, Meyer T, Stryer L. Range of messenger action of calcium ion and inositol 1,4,5-trisphosphate. Science 1992; 258:1812-1815.
58. Baimbridge KG, Celio MR, Rogers JH. Calcium-binding proteins in the nervous system. Trends Neurosci 1992; 15:303-308.
59. Kasai H, Petersen OH. Spatial dynamics of second messengers: IP_3 and cAMP as long-range and associative messengers. Trends Neurosci 1994; 17:95-100.
60. Leckie C, Empson R, Becchetti A et al. The NO pathway acts late during the fertilization response in sea urchin eggs. J Biol Chem 2003; 278:12247-12254.
61. Raymond CR, Redman SJ. Spatial segregation of neuronal calcium signals encodes different forms of LTP in rat hippocampus. J Physiol 2006; 570:97-111.
62. Berridge MJ, Lipp P, Bootman MD. The versatility and universality of calcium signalling. Nat Rev Mol Cell Biol 2000; 1:11-21.
63. Parekh AB, Putney JW Jr. Store-operated calcium channels. Physiol Rev 2005; 757-810.
64. Tsien RY. Fluorescent probes of cell signaling. Annu Rev Neurosci 1989; 12:227-253.
65. Myiawaki A, Llopis J, Heim R et al. Fluorescent indicators for Ca^{2+} based on green fluorescent proteins and calmodulin. Nature 1997; 388:882-887.
66. Brundage RA, Fogarty KE, Tuft RA et al. Calcium gradients underlying polarization and chemotaxis of eosinophils. Science 1991; 254:703-706.
67. Laffafian I, Hallett MB. Does cytosolic free Ca^{2+} signal neutrophil chemotaxis in response to formylated chemotactic peptide? J Cell Sci 1995; 108:3199-3205.
68. Xu HT, Yuan XB, Guan CB et al. Calcium signaling in chemorepellant Slit2-dependent regulation of neuronal migration. Proc Natl Acad Sci USA 2004; 101:4296-4301.
69. Blaser H, Reichman-Fried M, Castanon I et al. Migration of zebrafish primordial germ cells: a role for myosin contraction and cytoplasmic flow. Dev Cell 2006; 11:613-627.
70. Kater SB, Mattson MP, Cohan C et al. Calcium regulation of the neuronal growth cone Trends Neurosci 1988; 11:315-321.
71. Gomez TM, Zheng JQ. The molecular basis for calcium-dependent axon pathfinding. Nat Rev Neurosci 2006; 7:115-125.
72. Robles E, Huttenlocher A, Gomez TM. Filopodial calcium transiente regulate growth cone motility and guidance through local activation of calpain. Neuron 2003; 38:597-609.
73. Henley JR, Huang KH, Wang D et al. Calcium mediates bidirectional growth cone turning induced by myelin-associated glycoprotein. Neuron 2004; 44:909-916.
74. Wen Z, Guirland C, Ming GL et al. A CaMKII/calcineurin switch controls the direction of Ca^{2+}-dependent growth cone guidance. Neuron 2004; 43:835-846.
75. Schmidt JT, Morgan P, Dowell N et al. Myosin light chain phosphorylation and growth cone motility. J Neurobiol 2002; 52:175-188.
76. Wayman GA, Kaech S, Grant WF et al. Regulation of axonal extension and growth cone motility by calmodulin-dependent protein kinase I. J Neurosci 2004; 24:3786-3794.
77. Tang F, Kalil K. Netrin-I induces axon branching in developing cortical neurons by frequency-dependent calcium signalling pathways. J Neurosci 2005; 25:6702-6715.
78. Lautermilch NJ, Spitzer NC. Regulation of calcineurin by growth cone calcium waves controls neurite extension. J Neurosci 2000; 20:315-325.
79. Dawson TM, Sasaki M, Golzales-Zulueta M et al. Regulation of neuronal nitric oxide synthase and identification of novel nitric oxide signalling pathways. Prog Brain Res 1998; 118:3-11.
80. Aspenstrom P. Integration of signalling pathways regulated by small GTPases and calcium. Biochem Biophys Acta 2004; 1742:51-58.
81. Fleming IN, Elliott CM, Buchanan FG et al. Ca^{2+}/calmodulin-dependent protein kinase II regulates Tiam1 by reversible protein phosphorylation. J Biol Chem 1999; 274:12753-12758.
82. Price LS, Langeslag M, ten Klooster JP et al. Calcium signalling regulates translocation and activation of Rac. J Biol Chem 2003; 278:39413-39421.
83. Woo S, Gomez TM. Rac1 and RhoA promote neurite outgrowth through formation and stabilization of growth cone point contacts. J Neurosci 2006; 26:1418-1428.
84. Broussard JA, Webb DJ, Kaverina I. Asymmetric focal adhesion disassembly in motile cells. Curr Opin Cell Biol 2008; 20:85-90.
85. Ezratty EJ, Partridge MA, Gundersen GG. Microtubule-induced focal adhesion disassembly is mediated by dynamin and focal adhesion kinase. Nat Cell Biol 2005; 7:581-590.
86. Panicker AK, Buhusi M, Erickson A et al. Endocytosis of beta1 integrins is an early event in migration promoted by the cell adhesion molecule L1. Exp Cell Res 2006; 312:299-307.
87. Ooashi N, Futatsugi A, Yoshihara F et al. Cell adhesion molecules regulate Ca^{2+}-mediated steering of growth cones via cyclic AMP and ryanodine receptor type 3. J Cell Biol 2005; 170:1159-1167.

88. Itoh K, Stevens B, Schachner M et al. Regulated expression of the neural cell adhesion molecule L1 by specific patterns of neural impulses. Science 1995; 270:1369-1372.
89. Hanson MG, Landmesser LT. Normal patterns of spontaneous activity are required for correct motor axon guidance and the expression of specific guidance molecules. Neuron 2004; 43:687-701.
90. Nishimune H, Sanes JR, Carlson SS. A synaptic laminin-calcium channel interaction organizes active zones in motor nerve terminal. Nature 2004; 432:580-587.
91. Sann SB, Xu L, Nishimune H et al. Neurite outgrowth and in vivo sensory innervation mediated by a $Ca_V2.2$-laminin β2 stop signal. J Neurosci 2008; 28:2366-2374.
92. Jacques-Fricke BT, Seow Y, Gottlieb PA et al. Ca^{2+} influx through mechanosensitive channels inhibits neurite outgrowth in opposition to other influx pathways and release from intracellular stores. J Neurosci 2006; 26:5656-5664.
93. Brackenbury WJ, Davis TH, Chen C et al. Voltage-gated Na^+ channel β1 subunit-mediated neurite outgrowth requires Fyn kinase and contributes to postnatal CNS development in vivo. J Neurosci 2008; 28:3246-3256.
94. Grimes JA, Fraser SP, Stephens GJ et al. Differential expression of voltage-activated Na^+ currents in two prostatic tumour cell lines: contribution to invasiveness in vitro. FEBS Lett 1995; 369:290-294.
95. Diss JK, Fraser SP, Djamgoz MB. Voltage-gated Na^+ channels: multiplicity of expression, plasticity, functional implications and pathophysiological aspects. Eur Biophys J 2004; 33:180-193.
96. Comoglio PM, Trusolino L. Cancer: the matrix is now in control. Nat Med 2005; 11:1156-1159.
97. Girieca L, Ruegg C. The tumor microenvironment and its contribution to tumor evolution toward metastasis. Histochem Cell Biol 2008; 130:1091-1103.
98. Bhowmick NA, Moses HL. Tumor-stroma interactions. Curr Opin Genet Dev 2005; 15:97-101.
99. Ferrara N, Gerber HP, LeCouter J. The biology of VEGF and its receptors. Nat Med 2003; 9:669-676.
100. Radisky DC, Levy DD, Littlepage LE et al. Rac1b and reactive oxygen species mediate MMP-3-induced EMT and genomic instability. Nature 2005; 436:123-127.
101. List K, Szabo R, Molinolo A et al. Deregulated matriptase causes ras-independent multistage carcinogenesis and promotes ras-mediated malignant transformation. Genes Dev 2005; 19:1934-1950.
102. Stefanidakis M, Koivunen E. Cell-surface association between matrix metalloproteinases and integrins: role of the complexes in leukocyte migration and cancer progression. Blood 2006; 108:1441-1450.
103. Fidler IJ. The pathogenesis of cancer metastasis: the 'seed and soil' hypothesis revisited. Nat Rev Cancer 2003; 3:453-458.
104. Weinberg RA. The Biology of Cancer. Garland Science, New York: 2006.
105. Maher EA, Furnari FB, Bachoo RM et al. Malignant glioma: genetics and biology of a grave matter. Genes Dev 2001; 15:1311-1333.
106. DeAngelis LM. Chemotherapy for brain tumors—A new beginning. N Engl J Med 2005; 1036-1038.
107. Lefranc F, Brotchi J, Kiss R. Possible future issues in the treatment of glioblastomas: special emphasis on cell migration and the resistance of migrating glioblastoma cells to apoptosis. J Clin Oncol 2005; 23:2411-2422.
108. Stupp R, Mason WP, van den Bent MJ et al. European organisation for research and treatment of cancer brain tumor and radiotherapy groups radiotherapy plus concomitant and adjuvant temozolomide for glioblastoma. N Engl J Med 2005; 352:987-996.
109. Giese A, Bjerkvig R, Berens ME et al. Cost of migration: invasion of malignant gliomas and implications for treatment. J Clin Oncol 2003; 21:1624-1636.
110. Lefranc F, Kiss R. The sodium pump α1 subunit as a potential target to combat apoptosis-resistant glioblastomas. Neoplasia 2008; 10:198-206.
111. Olsen ML, Sontheimer H. Voltage activated ion channels in glial cells. In: Ransom BR, Kettenmann H, eds. Neuroglia. Oxford:Oxford University Press, 2005.
112. Kimelberg HK, Macvicar BA, Sontheimer H. Anion channels in astrocytes: biophysics, pharmacology and function. Glia 2006; 54:747-757.
113. Theodosis DT, Poulain DA, Oliet SHR. Activity-dependent structural and functional plasticity of astrocyte-neuron interactions. Physiol Rev 2008; 88:983-1008.
114. Papadopoulos MC, Saadoun S, Verkman AS. Aquaporins and cell migration. Pflugers Arch 2008; 456:693-700.
115. Bordey A, Sontheimer H. Postnatal development of ionic currents in rat hippocampal astrocytes in situ. J Neurophysiol 1997; 78:461-477.
116. MacFarlane SN, Sontheimer H. Changes in ion channel expression accompany cell cycle progression of spinal cord astrocytes. Glia 2000; 30:39-48.
117. Kofuji P, Ceelen P, Zahs KR et al. Genetic inactivation of an inwardly rectifying potassium channel (K_{ir} 4.1 subunit) in mice: phenotypic impact in retina. J Neurosci 2000; 20:5733-5740.

118. Olsen ML, Hishigamori H, Campbell SL et al. Functional expression of K_{ir} 4.1 channels in spinal cord astrocytes. Glia 2006; 53:516-528.
119. Chittajallu R, Chen Y, Wang H et al. Regulation of K_v1 subunit expression in oligodendrocyte progenitor cells and their role in G1/S phase progression of the cell cycle. Proc Natl Acad Sci USA 2002; 99:2350-2355.
120. Higashimori H, Sontheimer H. Role of K_{ir} 4.1 channels in growth control of glia. Glia 2007; 55:1668-1679.
121. Olsen ML, Schade S, Lyons SA et al. Expression of voltage-gated chloride channels in human glioma cells. J Neurosci 2003; 23:5572-5582.
122. Olsen ML, Weaver AK, Ritch PS et al. Modulation of glioma BK channels via erbB2. J Neurosci Res 2005; 81:179-189.
123. Ross SB, Fuller CM, Bubien JK et al. Amiloride-sensitive Na^+ channels contribute to regulatory volume increases in human glioma cells. Am J Physiol Cell Physiol 2007; 293:C1181-C1185.
124. Masi A, Becchetti A, Restano-Cassulini R et al. hERG1 channels are overexpressed in glioblastoma multiforme and modulate VEGF secretion in glioblastoma cell lines. Brit J Cancer 2005; 93:781-792.

INDEX

A

Actin cytoskeleton 5, 43, 45, 46, 48, 49, 107-111, 114
Activation 1-5, 10, 13, 15, 16, 18, 19, 24, 30, 40, 43-52, 58-62, 64, 69-74, 76, 77, 81, 84, 85, 87-89, 95, 98-102, 108, 109, 111, 112, 116, 118
Adherence 81, 84
Adhesion point 109, 110, 114
Affinity-based technology 25, 26, 30
Antiarrhythmic drug 58
Arginine-glycine-aspartic acid (RGD) sequence 3, 27, 30, 40, 43, 44, 70, 71, 73, 76, 77, 98-100
Aspecific interaction 28

B

Biochemical approach 30, 38, 40
Bone marrow 58, 62, 85, 116

C

Ca^{2+} channel 2, 11, 17, 18, 69-72, 76, 100, 111, 113, 115
Ca^{2+} signaling 74, 113-115
Calcium-activated potassium (BK) channel (Ca^{2+}-activated K^+ channel) 15, 69, 74-77, 114, 124
Cancer 31, 41, 49, 51, 52, 55, 56, 58, 59, 61, 64, 65, 84, 101, 115, 116
Cell activation 40
Cell differentiation 55, 58, 59, 62
Cell migration 6, 45-51, 58, 61, 64, 107-113, 115, 118
Cell proliferation 17, 47, 50, 51, 55, 56, 58, 59, 62, 64, 102, 118
Channel blocker 56, 64
Cl^- channel 5, 17, 18, 56, 124
Co-immunoprecipitation 24, 38, 49, 61
Colorectal cancer 58, 59, 61, 64
Conformational coupling 30, 55, 64
Cortical synapse 96

Cross-linking 28-30, 74, 108
CXCR4 62-64
Cyan fluorescent protein (CFP) 35, 39-41

D

Deactivation 10, 13
Delayed rectifier K^+ current 16
Desensitization 9-11, 13
Developing and adult brain 96

E

EGF receptor (EGFR) 40, 41, 48, 49, 51
Endothelium 5, 70, 74
Epileptogenesis 95, 98
Epitope 26, 27, 40, 64, 65
Extracellular matrix (ECM) 1-5, 43, 44-52, 55, 59, 69, 70, 72, 74, 76, 77, 81, 84, 96, 98, 102, 109, 111, 114, 116

F

Far Western Blot Analysis (Far WB) 25, 29
Fibronectin 2, 43, 49, 59, 69-72, 89, 96, 101, 102
Fluorescence lifetime imaging microscopy (FLIM) 33, 36, 37, 40, 41
Fluorescence microscopy 33, 34, 38
Fluorescent antibody 33, 34, 39
Fluorescent fusion protein 33
Focal adhesion kinase (Faks) 43, 46-48, 50-52
Förster resonance energy transfer (FRET) 4, 33-41, 61, 113
Functional interaction 24, 55

G

Glioma 118
Glutamate receptor 5, 11, 18, 19, 95, 98-102
Green fluorescent protein (GFP) 33-35, 39, 40
Growth cone 100, 107, 109, 110, 113, 115

H

hERG 5, 6, 13, 15, 27, 28, 33, 35, 41, 55-64, 74, 118
High-throughput analysis 23, 26, 29

I

ILK 45, 50, 51
Integrin 1-5, 6, 9, 13, 15, 16, 18, 19, 23, 24, 26-30, 33, 35, 40, 41, 43-52, 55, 56, 59-64, 69-77, 81, 84-89, 92, 95-102, 107, 109-112, 115
Integrin signaling 4, 13, 40, 43, 44, 46, 51, 52, 69, 99
Integrin structure 1, 2, 43
Intracellular signaling 3, 11, 18, 43, 46, 55, 64, 76, 102
Invasiveness 55, 64, 107, 116, 118
In vitro 6, 23, 26-28, 51, 56, 62, 64, 81, 115
Inwardly rectifying K^+ channel (IRK) 13, 16, 84, 85, 86, 111, 112, 118
Ion channel 1, 5, 9-11, 13, 14, 18, 19, 23, 24, 26-30, 33, 35, 40, 41, 55, 56, 59, 61-64, 70, 72, 76, 95, 96, 98, 100-102, 107, 111, 112, 115, 117, 118

K

K^+ channel 16, 27, 28, 33, 40, 56, 60, 69, 70, 73, 74, 81, 89, 92, 107, 111, 114, 118, 124
Keratinocyte 95, 100, 101, 112
Kir2.1 82-87
Kv1.3 5, 41, 86-91
Kv1.5 89, 91

L

Label transfer 28, 29
Leukemia 5, 6, 57-60, 62, 64
Ligand-gated channel 10, 11, 13, 18, 95, 96, 100, 113
Lipid raft 61, 62
Lipopolysaccharide 83, 84, 86
Long-term potentiation 98-100

M

Macromolecular complex 52, 55, 61-63
Macrophage 81-92, 116

Matricryptic site 76, 77
Matricryptins 77
Metastasis 49, 51, 52, 116, 118
Microfilament 108-110, 112, 118
Microglia 89
Migration 2, 6, 23, 45-51, 58, 61, 62, 64, 89, 96, 101, 107-115, 117, 118
Monocyte 46, 81, 82, 84-92
Mononuclear phagocyte 81, 82, 90, 92
Myogenic tone 69, 70

N

Nernst equation 10
Neurite extension 109, 113, 114
Neuroblastoma 27, 57-60, 62, 87
Neuromuscular junction (NMJ) 95, 100, 102, 115
Nicotinic acetylcholine receptor (nAChR) 9, 10, 13, 14, 18, 19, 100-102, 112
N-methyl-D-aspartate (NMDA) 5, 18, 19, 98, 99

O

Outwardly rectifying K^+ (Kdr) current 13, 74, 81, 84, 86-90

P

p130Cas 46-48, 50, 51
p140Cap 47
Patch-clamp 2, 9, 10, 13, 19, 71, 81
Per-Arnt-Sym (PAS) domain 15, 56, 57, 61
Peripheral blood (PB) 58, 81-84, 87-90
Peritoneal 81-84, 88, 90, 91
Phagocytosis 89, 90
Photoaffinity labeling 23-25, 28, 29
Physical interaction 24, 27, 30, 60
Potassium channel *see* K^+ channel
Protein array 24-26, 29
Protein-protein interaction 3, 23, 24, 26-30, 33, 34, 39-41, 44, 47, 57, 61
Pull-down assay 25, 27, 28, 30

R

Rectification 11, 13, 16, 111
Resting potential 18, 58, 118
Rho 46, 48, 107, 109-111, 114, 115

Index

S

SDS-PAGE 27, 29, 30
Signal transduction 3, 30, 43, 46, 50
Site-directed mutagenesis 23, 69, 72
Src 4, 5, 30, 40, 41, 43, 46-48, 50, 51, 60, 69, 71, 72, 74-76, 96, 99-111
Stable protein-protein interaction 28
Synaptic plasticity 98, 100, 102, 108
Synaptogenesis 95, 96, 98, 102

T

Total internal reflection fluorescence microscopy (TIRFM) 33, 35, 38, 40, 41, 61
Transient protein-protein interaction 28, 30
Tumor microenvironment 115
Tumor necrosis factor (TNF) 83, 89, 91
Tumor stroma 116

V

Vascular cell adhesion molecule-1 (VCAM-1) 2, 82-88, 90
Vascular smooth muscle (VSM) 5, 69-73, 75-77
VEGF receptor 1 (Flt-1) 62, 64
Very late antigen-4 (VLA-4) 83, 84
Voltage-gated Ca^{2+} channel 2, 11, 17, 18, 100, 113, 115
Voltage-gated K^+ channel 5, 9, 13-15, 56, 118
Voltage-gated L-type calcium channel 76

W

Wound healing 1, 107, 108, 112

Y

Yeast two hybrid screening 24
Yellow fluorescent protein (YFP) 35, 39-41